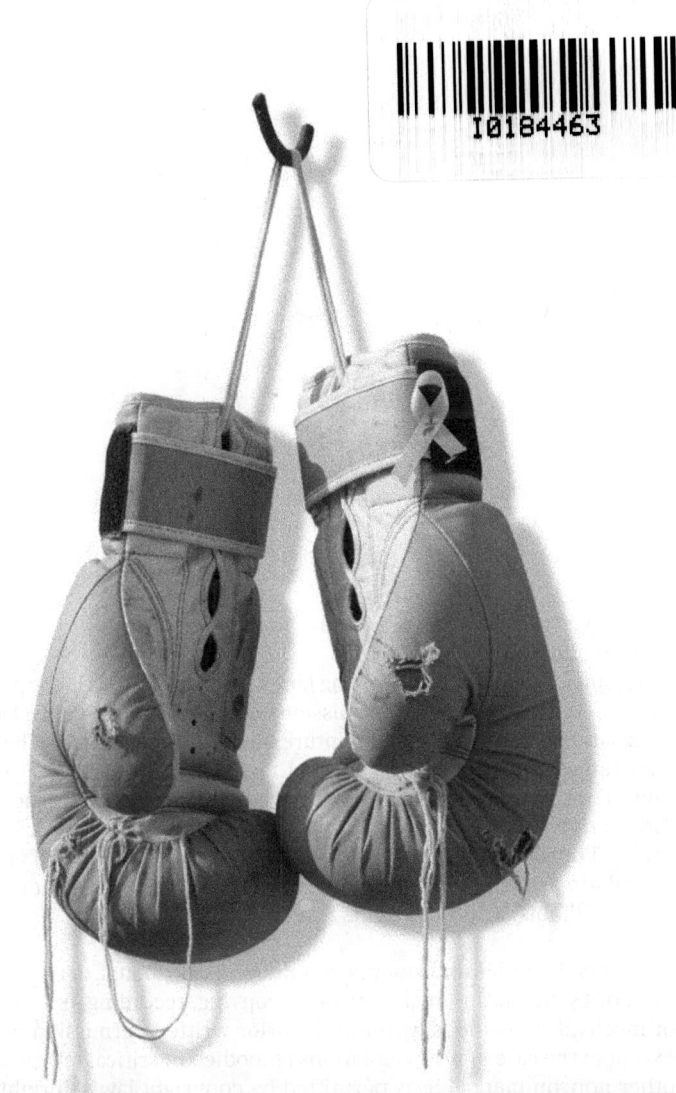

MAKING FAITH MOVES, NO MATTER WHAT

— A Memoir of Survival and Strength —

CASSANDRA L. REED

Copyright © 2026 Cassandra Reed
All rights reserved.
King James Version (KJV) The King James Version (KJV) is in the public domain and does not require special permission for use. Copyright: Public Domain. New International Version (NIV) Scripture quotations taken from The Holy Bible, New International Version®, NIV®. Copyright © 1973, 1978, 1984, 2011 by Biblica, Inc.® Used by permission. All rights reserved worldwide. New Living Translation (NLT) Scripture quotations are taken from the Holy Bible, New Living Translation, copyright © 1996, 2004, 2007, 2013 by Tyndale House Foundation. Used by permission of Tyndale House Publishers, Inc., Carol Stream, Illinois 60188. All rights reserved.

No part of this publication may be reproduced, distributed, or transmitted in any form or by any means, including photocopying, recording, or other electronic or mechanical methods, without the prior written permission of the author, except in the case of brief quotations embodied in critical reviews and certain other noncommercial uses permitted by copyright law. All rights reserved. For permission requests, please email the author at the address listed below.

Making Faith Moves No Matter What
A Memoir of Survival and Strength

Cassandra L. Reed
info@cassandralreed.com
cassandralreed.com

ISBN: 979-8-9938505-0-4
Printed in the United States of America

Cover and Interior Design by
Destined To Publish | Flossmoor, Illinois
www.DestinedToPublish.com

CONTENTS

Foreword

vii

Prologue

xi

Part I

My Three Son-Shines: My First Miracles and a Blessing

xxi

Chapter 1

Alice Walker: "Healing begins where the wound was made."

1

Chapter 2

Lauryn Hill: "Let me be patient, let me be kind, make me unselfish without being blind."

24

Chapter 3

Amiri Baraka: "Hope is delicate suffering."

30

Chapter 4

Maya Angelou: "When someone shows you who they are, believe them the first time."

44

Chapter 5

Rakim: "Constant elevation causes expansion."

49

Chapter 6

Tupac: "So no matter how hard it gets, stick your chest out, keep ya head up...and handle it."

68

Chapter 7

Notorious B.I.G.: "We can't change the world until we change ourselves."

88

Part II

The Degree – The Miseducation of Sandy, Using my Faith to Escape Poverty

Chapter 8

Malcolm X: "Education is our passport to the future, for tomorrow belongs to the people who prepare for it today."

97

Chapter 9

Gwendolyn Brooks: "Do not desire to fit in. Desire to oblige yourselves to lead."

116

Chapter 10

Nikki Giovanni: "Mistakes are a fact of life: It is the response to the error that counts."

123

Chapter 11
Jay Z: "Everybody can tell you how to do it, but they never done it."
131

Chapter 12
Langston Hughes: "The only way to get a thing done is to start to do it, then keep on doing it, and finally you'll finish it."
138

Part III
The Cancer—What Doesn't Kill You Makes You Stronger

Chapter 13
James Baldwin: "Love is a battle; love is a war; love is a growing up."
149

Chapter 14
Toni Morrison: "You wanna fly, you got to give up the sh*t that weighs you down."
163

Chapter 15
Nas: "Turnin' nothin' into somethin' is God work, and you get nothin' without struggle and hard work."
185

Chapter 16
Kendrick Lamar: "So next time you feel like your world is about to end, I hope you studied because He's testing your faith again."
192

Chapter 17

Zora Neale Hurston: "If you are silent about your pain, they'll kill you and say you enjoyed it."

199

Chapter 18

Oliver Wendell Holmes: "What lies behind us and what lies before us are tiny matters compared to what lies within us."

203

Epilogue by Joseph L Reed

A Journey of Love, Faith, and Strength from a husband's perspective

213

Acknowledgements

219

FOREWORD

"What is there possibly left for us to be afraid of, after we have dealt face to face with death and not embraced it? Once I accept the existence of dying, as a life process, who can ever have power over me again?" – Audre Lorde, The Cancer Journals

I've been thinking a lot about legacy - what it means, how we build it, and what I want to leave in the world when I become an Ancestor. In the face of multiple wars, genocides, spiritual and psychological attacks, fights for bodily autonomy and reproductive justice, and struggles for Black liberation across the globe, finding our unique purpose can feel daunting. We ingest the ills of the world - literally and figuratively - through the poisoned foods we eat, the toxins in the air we breathe, and the persistent dysregulation of our nervous systems as we navigate the contradictions of life in an oppressive, racial capitalist society. These ills find a home in our bodies and metastasize, sometimes in the form of cancer. For one in eight women, this cancer will manifest in our breasts.

It is likely unsurprising that this diagnosis has grave consequences for Black women. Consider these statistics: The American Cancer Society reports that Black women are two times more likely than White women to be diagnosed with Triple Negative Breast Cancer, one of the most aggressive and deadly forms of breast cancer. Additionally, even though Black women are diagnosed with breast cancer at similar rates as White women, Black women are 40% more likely to die from the disease due to a significant lack of access to quality healthcare and life-saving treatments. In fact, Black women have the lowest five-year relative breast cancer survival rate of all racial and ethnic groups. So, when Black women evoke our foremother, Fannie Lou Hamer's, infamous war cry, "I'm sick and tired of being sick and tired," we mean it quite literally.

Given the many ways our government and society perpetuate the disenfranchisement of oppressed peoples, it is vital that we remain steadfast in pursuing our legacy. The truth of the matter is that using one's gifts in service of our collective liberation in the temporary time we have on this earth is the only way we get free. So, we must be relentless in our pursuit to understand whether and how we are living in our purpose - naming for others what we hope our lives contribute to and for others.

Making Faith Moves, no matter what is a collection of reflections from a woman whose wisdom and purpose were sharpened by her experience with breast cancer. Cassandra Reed, my beloved cousin and soul sister, was diagnosed with cancer on April 23, 2021. Twelve years my senior, I have literally always looked up to her. And how could I not be in awe of her? Cassandra was this cool, smart, beautiful, and sassy woman who embodied the best parts of our foremothers but with a remix. We were raised on the South Side of Chicago by bold and brilliant Black women who poured a tremendous amount of love into us - love that was deep, pure, and complicated. Love for them was much more than a feeling; it was an ethic grounded in action. At the same time, it seemed as if the women who raised and loved us so well were not practiced at expressing that love toward themselves. Too often, love meant martyrdom to many women in our family. Love required a type of self-sacrifice that kept our foremothers in relationships and friendships that did not always honor the fullness of their needs and desires. Yet, I saw Cassandra attempt to do things differently; she strived to learn to love herself first.

When acclaimed poet Audre Lorde wrote the incredible book The Cancer Journals in 1980, she emphasized the significance of women using their voices to speak their truths rather than allowing fear to embolden their silence. She wrote, "I do not wish my anger and pain and fear about cancer to fossilize into yet another silence, nor to rob me of whatever strength can lie at the core of this experience, openly acknowledged and examined" (p. 9). Silence, albeit sometimes convenient, is a trap that keeps us separated from the fullness of ourselves, each other, and our purpose. Indeed, I can remember a time when Cassandra would have chosen silence – to bear the load of the physical, psychological, and spiritual tolls of her cancer journey alone. However, she decided differently then, and she's choosing differently now. Her decision to share her story in this book is an important lesson that self-care and self-preservation are not individual endeavors. Cassandra reminds us that these acts are undoubtedly communal acts that cannot be achieved to their fullest potential in isolation because we learn and heal better when we do so in beloved community. This is a lesson that so many of us desperately need to embrace.

To Sistas who have felt the weight of their own mortality, who have watched breast cancer and other illnesses ravage our bodies, who have had their spirits and hope crushed, who have fought hard to build a life their younger selves could have never imagined, this book is for you. By rejecting silence and despair in the face of life-altering challenges, Cassandra's life and words are a gift—a benediction to women everywhere on how to live in their legacies NOW with power, purpose, and deep conviction. May we all learn from Cassandra's stories and embrace the undeniable fact that it's our time to take back our power and build a legacy that reaches backward and forward – doing our part to create a world where we and our descendants can thrive in the fullness of their purpose.

In Eternal Hope & Struggle,

Dr. Aireale J. Rodgers

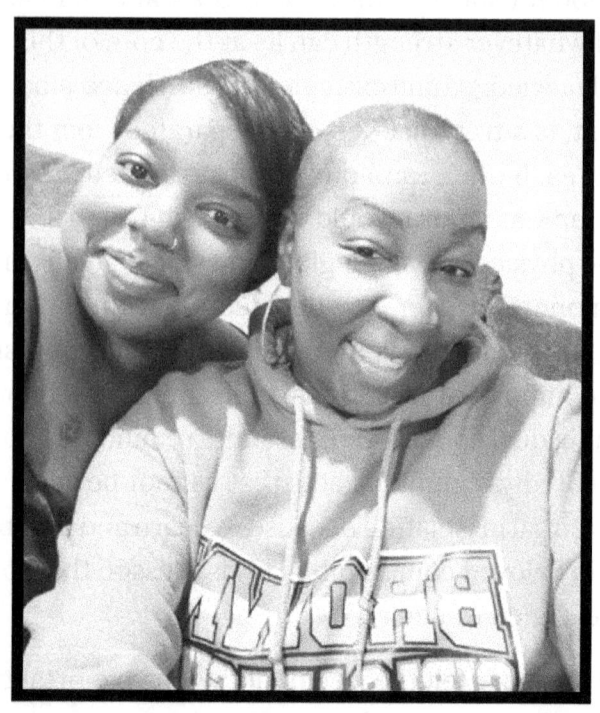

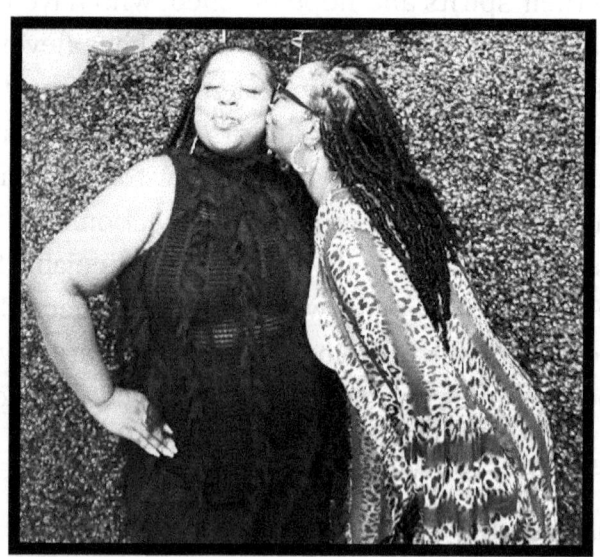

PROLOGUE

> I ran and ran and ran every day, and I acquired this sense of determination, this sense of spirit that I would never, never give up, no matter what else happened.
>
> Wilma Rudolph

In a relay race, each runner competes for both them and their team. The runner takes their mark and, with the word "Go," sprints into action, muscles tightening with each progression of the race. Adrenaline moves through the runner's body—so much that they become oblivious to anything around them. They hear no sounds; they only see their goal. Running around corners, knowing the precise time to slow down on the edges, feet up, knees bent, moving, heart pumping, getting the job done. I am not a runner; however, running is how I felt throughout my life as I faced many challenges.

Even when the runner fumbles, they don't stay down. They shake it off and get back on track. To get through the trials, you must stay motivated by conquering it and encourage yourself along your journey. Running hard and fast, keeping the momentum but pacing themselves as they see their teammates to whom they must pass the baton. Each teammate has a specific talent that assists the team in winning. The runner sends good thoughts to the teammates as they pass the baton—wishing them the best as they take off to complete the race. The effort is not singular; getting the gold medal is a team effort. Every runner's journey begins with a commitment to put one foot in front of the other continuously. Running demands a lot from your body, so be clear of your health before proceeding. Sometimes we run the 4 X 400-meter event, and other times it is for the long haul.

That is the first step to making a vow. That is a conscious choice to start the race. Mindset is powerful in achieving any goal, just like running. Stay focused on your goals and vision while remaining open to your greater purpose as you run.

I have experienced sexual abuse, poverty, grief, depression, abusive relationships, adultery, single motherhood with three Black, African American gentlemen, and Stage 2B triple-negative breast cancer. I am a person with many realities—I have experienced bad situations and bad relationships. I have been a liar and a cheater, and I didn't always make the best decisions. Yet, God is still using me to deliver a message. I am not a perfect person, but I serve a perfect God with faith and in truth on purpose. I live in my truth no matter how hard it gets. I have survived everything I was dealt with by facing it; I am still here. As the Bible says in Philippians 3:13-14, "No, dear brothers and sisters, I have not achieved it, but I focus on this one thing: Forgetting the past and looking forward to what lies ahead. I press on to reach the end of the race and receive the heavenly prize for which God, through Christ Jesus, is calling us." I cannot take credit for my triumph. It is indeed a gift from God. My faith in God was tried, tested, and prevailed every time I used Faith Moves and the agility and resilience I learned throughout my life. Faith Moves activate your inner confidence in God to move through life, even when you cannot see your next step. These are the lessons I share with you in this book.

Someone asked me: How did you make it through all your battles? My response? Faith! I used my faith in God to get me through all of it. As scripture teaches us, faith without work is dead. So, I had to do the work. I learned, for example, that over 200 muscles are activated in a single step while running. The endurance to run is work. Although I prefer brisk walking over running, using a relay race best illustrates how it felt to overcome my challenges.

No one gets through trauma and tragedies alone. I have been blessed with some wonderful family and friends who were my tribe through it all. They listened to me, prayed for me, affirmed me, and often advocated for me. Running a relay race cannot be won without a great team. Make sure those around you are encouraging, supportive, and willing to go the distance with you, fighting to win every step of the way.

My intention to share my story is to encourage and motivate someone who may have similar experience and is trying to figure it out. Here, I am sharing three of the toughest storms I walked through to illustrate how I succeeded because of my faith and my effort to do the work. You can, too. The three son-shines I gave birth to, the pursuit of my degrees, and my battle with cancer were three of my toughest battles, but they taught me to make Faith Moves no matter what.

As Claudia Tate states, "By and large, Black women writers do not write for money or recognition. They write for themselves as a means of maintaining emotional and intellectual clarity, of sustaining self-development and instruction. Each write because she is driven to do so..." I write for those very reasons as well as compassion for others facing challenging times. This book highlights my journey of trials, tragedies, and triumphs. In my journey of trying to achieve my undergraduate degree, I began naming my storms with scriptures. For example, Philippians 4:13 states, "I can do all things through Christ, which strengthens me," and this influenced the name I chose for my degree journey. Whenever I doubted myself or had bad days, I recited that scripture. I used Jeremiah 29:11 to get through my battle with breast cancer, "for I know the plans I have for you," declares the LORD, "plans to prosper you and not to harm you, plans to give you hope and a future."

I have been through some rough events, but I did not allow those incidents to make me bitter or cold. I sought guidance and direction. I reflected on the experience to understand its purpose and avoid repeating the same situation in the future. I kept my eyes on the hills. I take the high road instead of matching energy I choose distance. I held on to God for dear life, especially during my storms. In my experience, I find spiritual guidance and support within my faith community during times of personal challenge. In such moments, I view God as a source of healing and the church as a place of restoration, offering comfort and resilience when facing adversity.

Imagine your life, fighting obstacle after obstacle, all in the name of going after the ambitions you've set for your life. No one tells you that once you set goals for your life, you may face abuse, heartbreak, depression, and health issues along the way. You may feel you are all alone in the world, like no one sees your efforts or sees YOU. I have been there, and so I had to reveal my past hurt to heal. I had to go back and rescue the little girl I left at the sight of trauma. I had to take accountability for my actions and choices—both good and bad choices. I had to apologize for my toxic behavior. I had to make better decisions. I had to slow down. I had to learn how important my relationship with God is to do and be better. I had to stand in the mirror and examine my toxic traits and why they existed. I trusted God and sought therapy. I have reciprocal friendships that ensure we are our best selves. There is a safe space for growth and evolution without competition. I did this work on myself, making my inside beautiful, identifying more of God's characteristics and less of mine. I start my days with gratitude by reading a devotional/scripture, taking my vitamins, drinking my water, minding my business and hitting the ground running. I play my music beginning with gospel to hip hop to positive affirmations. I go to the gym for exercise and move my body for at least 30 minutes a day. I maintain boundaries and aim to preserve my well-being by avoiding negative behaviors or past situations I have moved on from.

Life is mostly about how you handle challenges, not just what happens to you. Whatever you have gone through, please believe it was not in vain. Turn it around for your purpose. When you stumble and fall, don't stay there, don't let that be the end of your story, pick yourself back up. Dr. Eric Thomas said it best when he wrote, "It's about getting up every day, understanding your power, walking in your purpose, knowing what you want, and spending every minute of the rest of your life going after it." If God gave you a testimony, use it to help someone else heal from what you have been through—that is the cheat code. You are indeed here for a reason. I beg you to find your God-given purpose and work towards achieving it until your last breath. This mission is personal. It takes a lot of strength to start over again time after time, but you owe it to yourself to become whatever you want and create the life you desire. Be brave. Go get it!

I became aware of discussions about me among individuals to whom I have demonstrated considerable support; however, they have formed perceptions that do not accurately reflect my character. What people think about you is not your business or your issue. It is theirs. Some people may dislike you because you are who they wish they could be. There are people who will despise you because of the way you shine, your aura and energy you bring. I played myself small for so long to make others more comfortable with me. I am no longer doing this. Trauma makes you feel as if you are responsible for other people's moods or behavior, so you work hard to make sure everyone feels good. I realize now that I worked hard to remove the "no" from people when it came to me. With any relationship in my life, whether family or friends, I became whoever I needed to be for that person, to make *their* lives better. I removed any reason anyone would want to tell me "No" by being a "yes" girl. I made myself so easy to love—so I thought. This tactic helped in my business life by making sure I had all the credentials and positive attitude necessary for any position I sought.

But when you are healed, you begin to realize it is not your responsibility how someone feels, acts, or behaves. You no longer attempt to manage the insecurities, wounds, or traumas of others. I focused on breaking generational trauma using my generational strengths from my ancestors and God. I am not only healing from the trauma I endured, but I am also healing from living my life in survival mode. For so long, I didn't know how to relax or enjoy a hobby. I preached to my children and myself for so long about doing what you *must* do until you can do what you *want* to do. While this thinking and mindset may have helped me elevate my career, it certainly did not help with my lack of emotional intelligence while raising my children. They had never seen me cry other than at church or a funeral. Back then, in my opinion, crying was a sign of weakness, and I was not weak. But I was so wrong. I have since apologized to my children for any trauma I caused them due to my ideologies at the time.

I absolutely love going walking it's been a form of meditation for me, and in my neighborhood along the trail, there is a hill I usually climb at the end of my walk before heading home. I was walking up this hill for exercise and looking at the ground on my way up, seeing all the insects and bugs. I saw the potholes and dog poop to avoid. While walking up the hill, I dodged all these objects I saw on my way to the top of the hill. That hill looked so intimidating from the bottom, as if the top was so far away and difficult to climb. I had to mentally decide if I wanted to climb the hill. Once my mind was made up to execute, my body followed. I climbed this hill one step at a time, regulating my breathing along the way. Being considerate of my endurance, I kept going. When walking up a hill, you experience an increase in altitude, also known as elevation gain. This refers to the total vertical distance you climb from your starting point to the highest point you reach. At the hilltop, the small distractions—like insects, bugs, or dog poop—were no longer visible or important. Once I reached the peak, the view from up high was so peaceful and serene. Even the air quality was different. I could inhale and exhale with ease at this elevation. The air was crisp and smelled fresh. Victory was mine because I did the work. Elevation can be seen as a process of rising above challenges and striving for a better version of oneself. It's about creating a more positive and fulfilling life by making conscious efforts towards personal growth. Researchers have found that experiencing elevation can lead to a more positive view of the world, increased spirituality, and a greater sense of meaning in life. I encourage you to keep rising to the top!

I am here today proclaiming that through it all, God saved me, and God will do the same for you. I tried doing it on my own and ended up abusing other vices (sex, dating, overworking, people-pleasing, and shopping) just to escape or ignore my problems. I am healed from the judgment of how I think, and I am healed from the grief of who I could have been had I never been traumatized. Smart people learn from their mistakes, wise people learn from the mistakes of others.

I am taking up space. I am presenting my experiences of overcoming adversity with the intention that they may provide motivation or insight to others. I am sharing my experiences transparently while using pseudonyms to protect the identities of individuals involved. My intention is to maintain confidentiality, avoid unnecessary conflict, and respect the privacy of all parties. I am sharing my story only, not to bash anyone.

Now I am the runner, and my children are my teammates, my legacy. I must give them everything I have before passing the baton to them to go further and farther than I could. I think about this book as a passing of a baton. Dear Reader, this book is for you to do the same. You, too, are my teammates. Let's run the race. Let's use our faith in God to make faith moves, no matter what. I won't tell you it will be easy because often it won't be. But it will be worth the effort. You are worth the effort.

The race is not given to the swift but to the one that endures to the end. Let's all start the marathon to see what lies at the finish line.

This book is respectfully dedicated to my ancestors who preceded me, my present family who supports me, and future generations yet to come.

If it doesn't challenge you, it won't change you.

FRED DEVITO

PART I

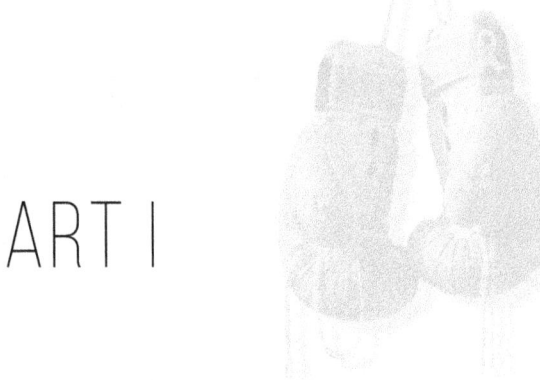

MY THREE SON-SHINES: MY FIRST MIRACLES AND A BLESSING

> *I'm not saying I'm gonna rule the world or I'm gonna change the world, but I guarantee you that I will spark the brain that will change the world.*
>
> **TUPAC AMARU SHAKUR**

But as it is written, Eye hath not seen, nor ear heard, neither have entered into the heart of man, the things which God hath prepared for them that love him.
1 Corinthians 2:9 KJV

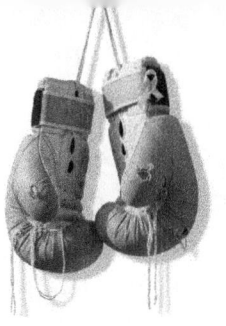

CHAPTER 1

Alice Walker:
"HEALING BEGINS WHERE THE WOUND WAS MADE."

I was born on June 19, 1976, and raised on the south side of Chicago, IL. My birthday is also known as Juneteenth. The National Museum of African American History and Culture traces Juneteenth's historical legacy back to "Freedom's Eve" on January 1, 1863, when the first Watch Night services occurred. On that night, enslaved and free African Americans gathered in churches and private homes across the country awaiting news that the Emancipation Proclamation had taken effect. At midnight, enslaved individuals in the Confederate States were legally declared free. Only through the Thirteenth Amendment did emancipation end slavery throughout the United States. But not everyone in Confederate territory would immediately be free. Although the Emancipation Proclamation took effect in 1863, it was not enforced in areas still held by Confederate authorities.

Consequently, in Texas, which was the westernmost Confederate state, the emancipation of enslaved people occurred later. On June

19, 1865, approximately 2,000 Union troops arrived in Galveston Bay, Texas, marking the official declaration of emancipation. The army announced that the more than 250,000 enslaved black people in the state, were free by executive decree. This day came to be known as "Juneteenth," by the newly freed people in Texas.

My father told me he used to sing "Isn't She Lovely?" by Stevie Wonder to me when I was a baby. I still play it every year on my birthday. My parents were both 20 years of age when I was born. They were young, they were fly, and both worked hard all my life.

I was the first daughter to my mother. When she was seventeen years old, she had my brother, Alonzo, with her first husband, Willie G, who we affectionately called "Moochie." Alonzo was 3 years older, and I was my father's first-born child, a daughter born a day before his first Father's Day. I'm one of three siblings: Alonzo, myself, and my younger sister Jeanette, who is two years younger than me. That makes me the middle child of my mother's children and the eldest of my father's children.

My mother, Helen, is the youngest child to her parents, Naomi and Charles. She has an older brother, my Uncle Gregory, and an older sister, my Auntie Bettye. After Naomi and Charles split up, my grandmother married Clarence, my second grandfather, who took us on memorable summer road trips down south.

My father, Eugene, was the first son to his parents. He has an older sister, Auntie Adrian, whom we affectionately called Auntie Agee. Then there was my aunt Cassandra (after whom I am named), but she passed away from crib death at about 3 months. Then came my father, Eugene—his first name is Elijah, like his own father, but he preferred using his middle name Eugene mostly). Then came the rest of the family: Auntie Sharon, Uncle Anthony (we called him Uncle Boobie), and Uncle Kimble who was about 10 years older than I was.

I always looked up to my mother from as far back as I can recall. She worked at a bank and dressed very nicely, always wearing nice heels, pretty dresses, light makeup, and hair always neatly set. She was classy and sophisticated but stern. She was my first role model. She was fierce and fine.

My father was my first best friend. He gave me attention, was easy to talk to and provided a safe space to share, took time to tell me how smart I was, and always celebrated my achievements, however small they were. The more he affirmed my success, the harder I worked to achieve success. I loved getting praise and hearing words of affirmation. My father loved the Cubs and used to take me to baseball games on my birthday, which usually fell on or around Father's Day every year. We both had a serious love of cookies and milk. I went to my father first about everything, even when I got my first menstrual cycle coming home from school. He took me to buy my first maxi pads and explained how to use them. When I was ready to lose my virginity, I told my father first, and he took me to the doctor to get on birth control pills. My father was easy-going, easy to talk to, and it didn't hurt that he spoiled me—not with possessions but with adoration. I always felt his love. I always felt he got me, and I understood him.

I was taught to respect others, avoid mocking people with disabilities or look differently, and not argue with adults. What I value most is seeing people treat others kindly. Many people poorly treat those they perceive as weaker, including the elderly, babies, and those with special needs. I regret having laughed at others when I was younger and less aware. As I've matured, I've learned to stand up against bullying and I support the underdog, regardless of popularity or trends. I don't follow trends or attach myself to people or brands just because everyone else does or because it's popular, this is something I learned as a child.

I greatly value spending time with my family, including my siblings, cousins, aunts, uncles, grandparents, and great-grandmother. Charles Berger is my mother's second cousin and closer in age to my parents than myself, he would sometimes take me to church with him by bus on Sundays. He consistently ensured my safety and took measures to protect me when I was with him. My cousin Charles is a big, dark-skinned black man from West Virginia, he talked fast and country. Some people don't take the time to understand what he is saying. I saw how people would make fun of him, belittle him and talk about him being illiterate. We created a special bond because I wanted to protect him and he also protected me, that remains to this day.

Cousin Charles, Uncle Boobie, and Uncle Tony used to live with us at different times when I was younger, and they all took good care of me. I have a special bond with them all for the extra care they have always given to me. I never felt invisible or unloved. My Uncle Jobe, who was married to my Auntie Sharon, was a favorite of mine, always welcoming and letting me know I could be anything I wanted to be. He always encouraged me to keep doing my best. My Uncle Gregory displayed the same love I received from all my uncles. In short, I always felt loved by my family and have always loved my family unconditionally. Especially the males in my family cherished us and told us we were pretty, gorgeous, smart—anything we wanted—and they showed nothing but love and respect. My aunts always cheered us on, whether we were excelling in school or dancing at a party. They all worked hard and played harder. I learned a lot from all of them, which shaped who I am today. My

Auntie Bettye taught me valuable life skills, style, to believe in myself and how to manage as a black woman. My Auntie Agee taught me to believe in myself and keep working hard in school to achieve no matter the obstacles. My Auntie Mimi taught me toughness, kindness, resilience and how to abound through every situation. My Auntie Sharon taught me how to enjoy my life and not care what anyone has to say. As I grew up, I always enjoyed spending time with each family member and lived to make my family proud.

Chicago in the 1980s was filled with great family memories. We were always surrounded by love. Both sets of grandparents partied together with the family every weekend. We usually gathered at my paternal grandparents' house in the Woodlawn area on 65th and Ellis (not sure of their exact address) every Friday night, and on Saturdays and Sundays after church. Woodlawn was a gregarious neighborhood on the South Side of Chicago, Illinois, near the shore of Lake Michigan, south of downtown, filled with mostly African American residents. I was brought up surrounded by family, who loved good food, good laughs, music, dancing, playing cards, and working hard. They were life-loving, God-loving folks. I learned manners from them: speak when I enter a room, respect my elders, stay out of adult business, and stay in a child's place. I was told to value education. I was assured that if I worked hard, I could be whatever I wanted to be.

My father especially was always reiterating the importance of education. If someone teasingly asked us girls in the family about having a boyfriend back then, my father's favorite advice was "Them books is your boyfriend." He always supported and encouraged the importance of education. I learned that it is best to have a positive outlook in life, and your character and attitude can take you a long way. I was taught not to lie. We couldn't even say the word "lie"; instead, we had to say, "You're telling a story." I learned how to carry myself outside our home because it reflected my parents and family. I never saw my mother step outside without looking her best, and that went for all the men and women in my family. I was taught to take pride in my appearance because, as I learned, you don't get a second chance to make a first impression.

I appreciated church and enjoyed going with my paternal great-grandmother Flora (her birth name was Dew Drop, but she didn't like it, so she changed it to Flora) to her church where she sang in the choir. I usually spent the night at her house with her and my Auntie Mimi, my paternal grandfather's sister, my father's aunt, and one of my favorite people. She advocates and defends me as fiercely as I do for her. I used to ride the 67th Street bus to 67th Ashland from 67th Paxton, where my great-grandmother's church was located. It was a small storefront type of church, filled with the singing of old hymns of praise. It was where I learned, "Jesus is on the mainline. Tell *Him* what you want." My great-grandmother used to lead the congregation, singing that song on many a Sunday. After church, I usually went to my paternal grandparents' house. My grandma Janet (pronounced Jeanette, my sister's namesake) would cook along with my aunts and mother. The men would usually be barbecuing, talking mess, gambling, playing records, or hanging out in the alley, but they could cook too, especially my father. My grandfather, Sonny Knox, made his own barbecue sauce that was so good, everyone came to visit looking for it.

My first cousins all grew up with me, most of us a year apart from one another. I grew up with so many first and second cousins that I couldn't name them individually, but I will say on 65th Ellis back in the 1980s, the family names were Knox, McNeil, Whitehead, Lymore, Thurmond, Smith, Love, Allen, Camp, Mitchell, Fisher, Sabbs, and

Richardson. We all fiercely protected each other, even though we teased each other relentlessly. Everyone knew our family on Ellis Avenue in Chicago, growing up in the Woodlawn area. As children, we played outside all day long until the streetlights flickered on. The men in our community fiercely protected us. We hung out at the playground and walked to the neighborhood candy store, which was often in someone's house. The candy store lady usually had penny candy, cookies, juices, pickles, and snow cones; it was all so good, you could throw a candy buffet for $1.00. We played Double Dutch with the jump rope—two people turned the ropes parallel but on opposite sides of each other to a regular beat, and at least one of us found the rhythm to jump inside the ropes to a made-up song. We also raced our bikes and big wheels up and down the neighborhood block, from one end to the next.

We girls made up cheers and performed the songs as we pumped our bodies and copied moves, we saw on television. Meanwhile, the boys participated in activities such as playing football or tossing a tennis ball against the wall and catching it upon its return, like racquetball. At the playground, we played on the swings, monkey bars, and seesaw—all tough metal embedded in concrete. In the past, playgrounds lacked rubber and other safety materials commonly used now. We played in dangerous conditions, unaware of the potential hazards. We waited for the ice cream truck to drive down our block and begged our parents for money to buy a succulent frozen dessert from the ice cream man. Once the streetlights came on, we headed back to our own homes. We raced each other to see who was the fastest.

Back at home, we played card games like Go Fish, War, Uno, and Spades. We made dances to songs like JJ Fad's "Supersonic" or Salt n Pepa's "Push It." We pretend-played school and church right in our house. We played "Rock Teacher" on the porch steps, a game where we guessed which handheld rock before we could advance to the next higher porch step. We cracked jokes on each other to see who could tolerate it or who would burst into tears. If you cried or got mad easily, we laughed until our bellies hurt. The lesson was: You had to toughen up. We fought each other physically and mentally but, at the same time, we were highly protective of each other. My family was upset when I didn't tell on my brother or cousin, but I stayed loyal regardless. No one outside the family was allowed to mess with any of us, or else they would be sorry.

I had my first fight when I was in the second grade at Alexandre Dumas elementary school with Ramona Hudson. I don't know why we fought but I remember afterwards we became the best of friends. If and when anyone outside our family touched me my brothers and male cousins would beat them up.

In the hot summer days back then, we turned on the fire hydrant in the neighborhood. Of course, that was illegal: Someone placed a block of wood or used a can open on both sides against the flow of water to pan it out or set their finger over the nozzle, so the water shot out like a fountain to cool us down. We threw each other into the spray, as cars would drive through cautiously or reverse-drive to avoid wetting their cars. This would persist until the fire department or police were contacted and arrived to stop the activity and turn off the water. We didn't have community centers or recreational play areas with swimming pools, so we had to create our fun with whatever was available. Summertime in Chicago in those days was so exciting for us, as he hung out with family at Rainbow Beach on South Shore Drive, played with siblings and cousins late into the night to catch lightning bugs in jars or holding them to our earlobes like earrings.

We spent summer evenings at our cousins' residences and met new people in their neighborhoods throughout the Southside. We went to the Taste of Chicago downtown around the Fourth of July to see the huge fireworks display. We didn't have a car among us, so we always took the CTA (Chicago Transit Authority) anywhere and everywhere.

My mother often took my siblings and cousins downtown on the CTA for movies or the Ringling Brothers' circus. Before summer ended and the school year began again, we all went to the Bud Billiken parade on the Southside at Washington Park and through Bronzeville on Martin Luther King Drive. Since 1929, the Bud Billiken parade is the largest African American parade held annually on the Southside the second Saturday in August and celebrates children returning to school. For the great event, my mother packed sandwiches and snacks in a cooler, and we carried blankets to sit on as we watched the parade. Carrying all this stuff made for an uncomfortably crowded bus ride sometimes, but we always enjoyed our effort to see the parade. We had to wake up early in the morning to catch the bus and find a good viewing spot so we could see all the acts perform—bands, dance groups, local celebrities, family and classmates performing in the parade. Our community consisted of dedicated families, with children in school and adults working, supporting one another through all circumstances. Although we had little money, we had a lot of love in our village.

We grew up living in poverty, but I never knew it until I went away to college. Even though we grew up walking to the laundromat pulling our cart with dirty laundry which we couldn't clean ourselves because we didn't have our own washer and dryer. But each generation tried to be better than the last one, to push our family and culture further and my parents were no exception. They did their best as providers and protectors. My parents provided us with more than they had while growing up, even though it wasn't necessarily with these tangible "luxuries." I am forever grateful for the hard work and sacrifices they made to raise me. Because of their love, support and hard work, it set the blueprint for my solid foundation.

I knew as a child that I wanted my life to be a little different—not better, but different. *The Cosby Show* was my favorite series back in the late 1980s, early 1990s. It depicted the successful Black family of a doctor married to an attorney raising four daughters and a son in New York. I was interested in pursuing a lifestyle similar to that depicted in *The Cosby Show* and becoming a lawyer like Claire Huxtable.

Back in the day, a Caucasian actress commented that *The Cosby Show* was fictional because a successful Black family like the Huxtables did not exist. I thought how wrong that was of her to speak about a race that wasn't hers, and I was determined to prove her wrong. Ironically, this same actress's show was cancelled after she made some racist remarks in 2023.

But with everything in life, there is ebbing and flow, right? I've mentioned all the joyful memories I had but, well, I also witnessed physical domestic violence in my family. I hated being woken by the sound of adults arguing and fighting. I couldn't sleep, couldn't rest, and always felt scared. I worked at trying to be unproblematic, the best child to make my family's life easier. I stayed clean instead of getting dirty when we played outside. I was an excellent student achieving good grades in school and faithfully attended church with my great-grandmother. These were the thoughts of a little girl who didn't understand that she could not control what other people did just by behaving herself. I made myself easy to love to ease the burden of others. In truth, I didn't fully understand or learn the lesson of this way of thinking until I was well past 30 years of age.

I can't remember for sure how young I was but based on where we lived at the time it happened, I was likely between 5 and 7 years old. I was molested. Twice—once at home, and once at my grandparents' home. This trauma changed my life forever. Once trauma takes hold, you can never retrieve the stolen innocence of a baby girl. I was robbed of giving away my virginity when I chose. I was robbed of my childhood. My body was now experiencing throbbing in a private place between my legs—a place I barely knew existed at my tender age. This was my first heartbreak but not the last. Now my mind, my thoughts, and my feelings no longer belonged to a little girl, but it forced me into an advanced emotional stage that I was ill-prepared for but had to endure.

Two separate events, two different people. I reassured myself by thinking it wasn't constant abuse. Because my family worked hard, they also partied a lot to offset it, and the merriment involved drinking, smoking, dancing, gambling, and talking mess, while the children were left to hang out in the back away from the grown people. I was one of the first girls born in the family of first cousins. It was mostly boys before me. Once again, I fiercely protect my family even against my own pain.

What did Sofia say in the movie "*The Color Purple*? "A girl child isn't safe in a house full of men." I was molested by two trusted family members on two different occasions. I didn't tell anyone because I didn't want to cause conflict. I didn't want them to get in trouble or be mad at me for getting them in trouble. They were not adults, I later rationalized, thinking they were not doing it to harm me. But they did it because they had free access to me as we were growing up, and their hormones were ruling their young bodies. Perhaps, as well, something had been done to them in their past. I forgave them and didn't tell anyone. It was not unusual as we grew up to play "house" and sometimes touch each other inappropriately.

However, the damage of these two specific episodes has followed me for the rest of my life in one way or another. I sometimes wonder why I felt it was up to me to protect everyone around me, even above myself and my pain. I was a child. I began to feel inner pain, a deep sadness inside. I started hurting myself by constantly picking at scabs that developed after I fell, and I would consistently peel the scab until it bled, no matter how much pain it caused. I sat and peeled and saw blood and did it again and again, alone in my room. I began to feel so ugly inside. I began to not like myself. I wanted to hide myself even from myself. In the outside world, I acted as if nothing had happened, but inside, I was torn apart. I abandoned the little girl I was and refused to defend her.

My parents separated around 1987. My father and uncle Boobie left Chicago to move down to South Carolina. That summer of 1987, my maternal grandparents drove me, my sister, and my cousins, Teneshia and Tinesha, on a road trip to South Carolina. We had a great time. We used to spend our days eating candy, making up dances to our favorite songs and raps, or heading to the swimming pool. My other cousins, Georgia and Carrie Jo, lived in South Carolina too, and we hung out with them to skate or join them on their paper routes. My great-aunt Renee and great-uncle Johnny lived in South Carolina too; Auntie Renee is my paternal grandmother's sister, and Uncle Johnny is her husband.

I noticed how dark people's skin would get from being beside the swimming pool in the summer. I wanted my skin to be a darker hue. By this time, I began having problem skin with acne. Because I habitually peeled my scabs and scars, I would burst the bumps on my face as well and pick at them. Because I was fair skinned, my face really looked bad from the damage, so I said, hey, if my skin was darker, people wouldn't see these marks on my face.

So, I decided I would sit by the pool and turn darker. I even defied my uncle's girlfriend, who told us to wait on Uncle Boobie before going to the pool, but I went anyway. I led my sister and cousins and myself straight to the pool, and we had a ball I intentionally sat outside the pool to darken my complexion and—to be honest, getting darker was also my way of fading into the background. I still felt terribly embarrassed and did not want to be seen ever since I had been molested. There I was, hiding myself in plain sight. I was forever changed and matured beyond my age. I also became my own worst critic because I felt as ugly as the thing others had imposed onto me. I now look back and saw how I began picking at pieces of myself that I didn't like…my physical appearance, my natural wavy hair. I wanted straight hair. I wanted to be darker and smooth-skinned. I didn't like my high cheek bones because I wanted dimples. I was a skinny girl with bony legs. I was self-sabotaging my outward appearance, and I wanted it to be on full display, even though I also wanted to disappear.

By the time I was in the sixth grade, my parents were together again but struggling so it didn't last long before they divorced and had new partners. (They were divorced by the time I started 9th grade.) We moved into the Burnside area from the Woodlawn area, which was still working lower-class. Burnside is one of the 77 community areas in Chicago. The 47th numbered area, it is located on the city's far south side. Our address was 651 East 92nd place. I was around 11 and my little sister was 9. Our older brother was a high school freshman, so he had to be at school earlier and didn't leave home at the same time as she and I did. Our parents left home on public transportation earliest of all of us. Our school was far from our apartment, so we walked when it was warm with a group of our friends, like the Nelson family, or we caught the CTA by ourselves to school when it was cold. The walk to school took about 15 or 20 minutes, but if it was too cold, we used our change to catch the bus which took less than half that time. Occasionally our classmates let us catch a ride to school with their parents.

Two CTA buses came to our stop—the 95th street bus (our bus) and the 4 Cottage Grove bus (the wrong bus). One time, we messed up and caught the wrong bus, and I had to comfort my little sister who became upset when it rolled straight on Cottage Grove instead of turning homeward to 93rd street. We were latchkey kids, which meant no one was home when we left for school or returned from school. My mother worked at a bank in downtown Chicago typically from 9 a.m. to 5 p.m., and her trek downtown was brutally long and crowded on the CTA. She had to leave early and didn't return home until we finished our homework. I remember my mother cooking dinner early in the morning before she left for work so we could warm it up in the oven ourselves and have a hot meal after school (she knew we wouldn't cook for ourselves—we were that lazy, but she was amazing!).

Our apartment was on the top floor of a building that looked like a single-family home with an addition on the roof—that is where we resided. Because our apartment was like an attic, all our rooms had slanted ceilings. We shared a three-bedroom apartment—our parents in one room, my brother in his own, and my sister and I in the third. We had a lot of fun in that neighborhood, although it was nothing like when we all lived in Woodlawn on Ellis, Greenwood, or Ingleside with our family. My friend Nicole was our next-door neighbor. When we first moved in, I noticed her playing in the street with some other girls and boys, dancing in short red shorts. I immediately thought she was a fast girl because she was so free in her moves in front of boys in her short shorts—we still laugh about that to this day.

In a new place, we had to make new friends outside of our family now. It was during this time that I met my lifelong friends: Maxine, Shantea, Ganell, Phenia, and Nicole. They are all still my sisters and brother. All my teachers at Oliver Hazard Perry were the bomb, in other words, good teachers. They were all Black, educated, sharply dressed, encouraging, take-no-mess teachers! How can you aspire to be a successful Black person without seeing representations of that around you? Representation matters. This fact wasn't missed on me at a time when we were constantly informed that successful, educated Black people simply didn't exist.

My sixth-grade teacher, Mrs. Holt, was a stout heavy-bosomed lady who wore her hair in a typically short and natural state. She always made up her face so nicely—she was gorgeous! My seventh/eighth grade teacher, Mrs. Wright, was also so beautiful. Her hair was always laid, bouncing, healthy. She wore beautiful suits, minimal makeup, loved her job. I also had Mrs. Pippion, Mr. Mays, and Mrs. Sorceby. Mr. Mays was the only male teacher I had, and he was tough. Of average height, he looked like he could have been a drill Sergeant in a past life. Smart, nicely dressed, good-looking. I always had a smart mouth, but I didn't play that with Mr. Mays. Whatever he said, I jumped to it. He could embarrass other classmates, and I did not want that treatment. One day, he told me to pass out the papers, but he called me by the wrong name. Looking dead at me, he said:

"Ann, come pass these papers out!"

I just stared, obliviously that he was talking to me.

Mr. Mays looked at me and this time yelled: "Ann, come pass out these papers!"

I jumped up from my desk and ran to get the papers from him to pass out. I didn't correct him on my name; I just did what he asked. For that whole day, I was Ann!

Growing up in the city, a kid is forced to grow up quickly. One day when I was around 12 years old, I walked to our local cleaners to pick up my mother's work clothes. It was empty except for the old Black man who worked there. He began acting weird with me, flirting, smiling, winking. Then, he offered to give me some money if I let him see my chest. He spoke while he tugged at the bottom of my T-shirt. I had bee sting-sized breasts, but until that moment, no one had ever mentioned my body in this way. I froze in place, scared to run or scream. Thankfully, two women entered the store, and I moved my feet right out that door. I went home and never told anyone about that until I was an adult in therapy. After that, I avoided doing errands at the cleaners or never went there alone. As my tiny breasts blossomed, men began noticing men who had watched me grow from a little girl to a pre-teen. They said provocative stuff as I walked through my neighborhood. "Hey shawty, you are looking good. Do you got a boyfriend yet, or I can teach you some stuff?"

A young girl roaming the big city must have a tough-as-nails exterior and a game face—no smiling, walking fast. Try to walk in groups. Don't go out alone at night, at least not without a weapon. My weapon of choice back then was a small box cutter, just mean enough to get someone off me. Thankfully, I had developed a tough exterior from my family roasting each other mercilessly as I grew up. When I went to college in Louisiana, people asked us Chicago people why we frowned and looked so mean. They always say Chicago girls have smart mouths and nasty attitudes. Well, as a

Chicago girl, I can say I learned this attitude early growing up and surviving the Southside. It was our defense mechanism. We're just built tough where I'm from.

One of the ways I coped and survived was through music. I fell in love with hip hop and rap music—what they called back in my day. I loved writing poems, short stories, and essays, so when I heard my brother blasting Eric B. and Rakim, Ice-T, King T, and other amazing artists, I got to know them well. I listened to Big Daddy Kane, MC Lyte, BDP, LL Cool J, Run DMC, Queen Latifah, NWA, and so many others that I still vibe out to today. I listened to a song once or twice and memorized all the words. People asked if I wrote the lyrics out to learn them so well. I laughed at that. No! Who has time for that? I would have to play it and then pause it to write down the lyrics then hit play again to listen more and write it down. Back in the day we had tape recorders!

Once, the boys in my class heard me rhyme all the words to "Don't believe the Hype" by Public Enemy, and they included me in their "boys club." I loved hip hop so much because those voices spoke up against injustice in our communities. I couldn't use my voice back then, so I buried myself in hip hop to speak for me. I loved the hard beats, the words, the clever way they worked together. How they used music to talk about our neighborhoods, to educate and motivate each other. This music was created by us and no one believed it would go worldwide. Critics said it wouldn't last, it would fade, in the 1970s. Fifty years later, it's still here and evolving and making so many wealthy and creating generational wealth for their families. I love an underdog; someone society has counted out and deemed unworthy. I could relate.

We rapped to the songs in the back of the school bus on field trips. We exchanged records with each other. I became like one of the guys—which made me feel safe to know that no one would sexually violate me if they saw me as one of them. So, I mostly hung with the guys—three during sixth through eighth grades: Anthony Payne, Darryl Jefferson and Larry Dean. Just as my father was my first best friend, these guys were my best friends at school. Rest in peace, Eddie Crisp—a good friend of mine with whom I graduated eighth grade, but he died in high school. That was one of the first funerals I attended for one of my classmates—and it wasn't the last, unfortunately. Losing friends to gun violence is just another way to grow up fast in the tough city. There are no children here. We faced the darkness of the world before we could even process a thought of who we were.

At thirteen, I began dating a guy named Jay who lived near my cousin's house. Jay was three years older than me. He was just about everything your parents warn you NOT to date. That didn't matter to me. He was tall, dark, and handsome, like one of my favorite rappers, Big Daddy Kane! Jay was my boyfriend from the time I was 13 until I turned 17—and I'll add that during most of that time, Jay was locked up in Cook County jail. I wrote him letters but never visited him. One summer when he was released from jail, I lost my virginity to him. I cringe at the mention of "virginity" because, in my view, my virginity had been taken from me when I was molested. Jay was very careful with my first time, taking time to love every part of my body. I was 16 years old; my sister and cousin Tinesha would tease me often because I was still a virgin, and I made Jay wait a long time before we had sex. Like I said, you can grow up fast in the city—most kids lost their virginity at the age of 12 or 13, or even younger.

I met one of my best friends, my sister friend Belinda, on the first day of freshman year. She was best friends with Nicole—another best friend who transferred from Perry and went to grammar school with Belinda. I used to eat lunch in my freshman year with people like Kim, Billie Jean, Pamela, Jafrika, and Belinda. I was a funny, cute, sometimes awkward, insecure, smart teenager. I had a decent wardrobe and fly hair and listened to nothing but hip hop. On my first day of high school, my brother Lonzo and cousin Terry walked me down the hall by the gym room where everybody hung out and announced that I was their little sister. They let everyone know not to mess with me. I was embarrassed but I felt their love and protection at that moment. People started calling me "Zo little sister" as if that was my name. Lonzo and Terry were both very popular on the football team. My brother was also on the track team and had been Prom King in junior year.

I remember walking back to school with Terry one day after cutting first and second period classes. As we approached the school, some boys in my class were throwing rocks in an open field. We walked through anyway, assuming they would stop throwing them, but they didn't. One rock hit my ankle. Terry was instantly enraged, cursed them out and chased them, even though they tried apologizing. I even felt sorry for them because Terry was a guy who fought very well. To be honest, they should have stopped throwing rocks! He protected me and handled them. As a result, I never feared anyone because I knew I had protection at any given time. If necessary, I could call someone in my family for assistance, and they would be there. Same as I would for them.

My first year of high school, my brother and cousin protected me. In my second year, I had my cousin. By my third year, I no longer had that protection because they both graduated high school and was away at college.

At sixteen, I was raped. I never told a soul for many years. Another secret of sexual abuse I kept to myself. Even though my family was close and loving, I still didn't feel like I could trust someone with that devastation. There were high expectations of me, and I didn't want to let anyone down. I blamed myself.

Around this time, my little brother, Elijah, was born to my father and his girlfriend, Yvonne. I loved this baby boy so much and took him with me wherever I went, mostly to my mom's house to babysit him and sometimes his sister—my stepsister, Ebony, who was a toddler when Elijah was born. I was fifteen and used to ride the CTA bus from my mother's house to pick him up from my father's house. The bus passengers commented that "my son" looked just like me. I just laughed and said, "I don't have any children. He's my little brother." People were so used to teenage pregnancy that they automatically assumed he was my son.

Family has always been very important to me. I believe in appreciating each person for who they are and what they add to my life. I don't believe one person can do everything, but everyone can do something. I can go to an aunt for a good recipe, or an uncle for self-defense tactics, a cousin for uplifting, or a sibling for financial knowledge. Just like baking a cake, you need different ingredients to come together to make something beautiful and delicious. I believe this same applies to your family or your village. Learn who you can go to for help because they have certain abilities to help get you wherever you need to go. In believing this, I never judge any of my family members for any of their shortcomings. I have learned to accept people for who they are and not for who I want them to be. That becomes unconditional love. Some people are better at supporting people emotionally, while others are best at financial support, and even still some may have a small capacity for physical support and that is it. No matter. We all must agree that everyone is passing through their own storms and face their own assignments and purpose from God. I understood the dynamic of family at an early age and moved through my life with much respect for my family, especially my elders. I always wanted to make my parents and elders proud and be a role model for those coming up behind me.

My Auntie Aggy used to play, "You Brought the Sunshine" by the world-famous Clark Sisters, and she taught me the song by singing it in my grandmother's kitchen while she cooked. I found comfort in seeing God as my Heavenly father watching over me, caring for me, and comforting me. God has always been my strength—that is one thing I trust without question. I love you, Lord; you are my strength (Psalms 18:1).

Making Faith Moves…There is a level of dysfunction in every family, and mine is no different. For sure, my good days have far outweighed my bad, including the trauma of being molested. Trauma is defined as a deeply distressing or disturbing behavior. Unhealed trauma can look like a low sense of self-worth, putting your needs aside for other people, and craving external validation. I have exhibited all these traits. I had to undergo a certain therapy style my high school friend who is a licensed therapist, Safiya, taught me, to free those words about being molested. I had severe body trauma recalling it because it had been suppressed for so long—and it still hurts. Trauma is real, and the stages of trauma are like the stages of grief. The first stage is denial, which looks like someone attempting to convince themselves nothing happened. I did this for years. My wound was made when I was molested. Those activities led me to begin a downward spiral in exhibiting low self-esteem. I had to rescue the little girl I left; I had to find her, defend her and affirm her to heal. Safiya also taught me how to do that, it involves putting your hand over your heart, closing your eyes, and communicating with the little girl internally crossing decades.

I read a quote on Instagram that read:

> Healing is so tough because it's a constant battle between your inner child, who's scared and just wants safety, your inner teenager who's angry and just wants justice, and your adult self, who is tired and just wants peace. Be gentle with yourself.

SWEET HOME CHICAGO

My Ode to Chicago.

I love my city, Chi-city, oh so pretty! Chicago was discovered by Jean Pointe Baptiste DuSable, a Haitian man. The Southside of Chicago is home for me and forever endearing to my heart. She is cold when necessary and warm when it's time. Every season is a vibe, and we put it on, from leather, suede, and furs to summertime Chi chilling on Lake Shore Drive watching Lake Michigan or boat riding along the river. She is smooth jazz, blues, stepping, gospel, dancing, house music, hip hop. We love music from all our local Chi-town artists. She is filled with entrepreneurs, educators, businessmen and women, fashionistas, and every career imaginable. We are built strong through these rough big city streets. We are gonna make it legally or illegally. Chicago is heart and pure soul.

I love my city, Chi-city, oh so pretty! Chicago is love, peace, and soul, like Don Cornelius said on *Soul Train* and equally gangster like Al Capone in *The Untouchables*. Our gangsters can perculate, step, do foot work and juke. She is filled with communities of hard workers, families, and freedom fighters. We fight for justice for all with the understanding that if Black Americans don't have justice here, no one else will. Rest in love LaQuan McDonald. Reverend Jesse Jackson and the Rainbow PUSH Coalition reside in Chicago along with Minister Louis Farrakhan, where you can see the crescent moon and five-point star high in the sky on Stony Island. Reverend Jeremiah Wright and Father Pfleger, who each have well-established platforms of equality, equity, and justice with their institutions of community service. We demand justice and peace for all in my city. Chicago ain't neva scared. My love spreads from the south side to over east, to outwest and up North.

I love my city, Chi-city, oh so pretty! Chicago presents a lavish and beautiful downtown bursting with skyscrapers, restaurants, culture, museums, art, and shopping. What city do you know is famous for popcorn, pizza puffs and mild sauce? She has every mode of transportation available every day 24 hours a day to get you anywhere in the city and surrounding suburbs. Chicago food is unmatched and available all hours of the day and night; any type you can name or desire of every ethnicity. Chicago has all the best sports franchises too! The Chicago Bulls, Chicago Sky, Chicago Bears, Chicago White Sox, Cubs, and Chicago Blackhawks, all winning teams. No other team did the Super Bowl shuffle like the 1985 Bears, and we loyally Bear down every football season in hopes of another Super Bowl. We enjoyed the back-to-back three-peat Bulls championships in the 1990s with a dream team led by Michael Jordan and Scottie Pippin. Chi City raised me and will be in my heart always. I am from Woodlawn, Burnside, 79th Colfax, east side crazy state to the lake. We wake up and just know, we can survive anything the day throws our way. Chicago is filled with champions.

I love my city, Chi-city, oh so pretty!

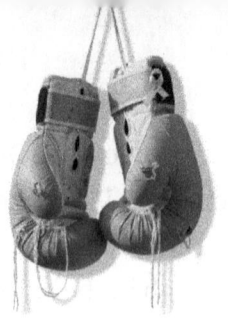

CHAPTER 2

Lauryn Hill:
"LET ME BE PATIENT, LET ME BE KIND, MAKE ME UNSELFISH WITHOUT BEING BLIND."

I met Mister in the cafeteria on the campus of Grambling State University in Louisiana during the second semester of my freshman year. He flirted, I flirted back, but I already had a boyfriend and told him as much. He wrote his dorm phone number on a piece of paper, gave it to me, and asked for mine. I was obliged, so we could talk on the phone. But I had no intention of talking to him after that day because I knew how jealous my boyfriend was, so I spent a lot of time with my boyfriend instead.

Eventually my boyfriend and I broke up because not having any space from him drove me crazy. I ended our relationship and began taking Mister's calls. We talked constantly. I learned he was born in Inglewood, California, graduated from Morningside High School, then moved to Monroe, Louisiana where his mother and grandparents lived. He was a psychology major—very smart; his grade point average was higher than mine. I was intrigued and attracted to his intelligence. He sometimes cooked and invited me over to hang with him and his family and friends off campus. I am a foodie, and he cooked well, so I was in love!

Our relationship began in March 1995. We took walks around campus. I adored looking at the stars at night and talking with Mister. When that semester ended in May, I was sad to leave Mister in Louisiana to go back home to Chicago for the summer.

We wrote each other letters and phoned constantly. The summer couldn't end fast enough for me to return to school in Louisiana to see Mister. We spent every chance we got together. I also started smoking marijuana with him. I wasn't as focused on school as I had been. My grades at the end of that semester reflected my poor performance. I ended up on academic probation. For one, I decided to stop the marijuana. Because I had no vehicle, I had to depend on friends to get anywhere off campus, so I decided not to return to school in the spring. Instead, I went home to Chicago to work so I could buy a car for school. That summer, Mister visited family in Michigan, not too far from Chicago, so I rented a car, and my cousin Tinesha and I went to visit him and stayed with my cousin Ida in Flint, Michigan. We hung out with Mister and his cousins, Tasha and Jeff. It was so good seeing each other again. The next semester, I went back to Grambling, found a job, and drove my own car. I was finally ready to get back on track in college.

This time, Mister dropped out to pursue a career as a rapper. He was in a group and managed by one of his good friends. They toured the southern regions of Louisiana and neighboring areas trying to make a name for themselves. At one point, a song from their album was played on the Top 8 songs of the week.

Right after the spring semester began in 1998, I found out I was pregnant. Mister and I had been dating for almost three years by now, so we were not as careful as we had been at the beginning of our relationship. We both got too comfortable, and I wasn't on birth control. Because I had never gotten pregnant before, I assumed I couldn't get pregnant since being molested and raped. I made up my mind that something was wrong with me. I never shared that thought with anyone, so when I took the pregnancy test, I was scared but excited at the same time. I had never been pregnant, and here I was 21 years old in college trying to get back on track, and-I was about to become a mother.

I always took a full class load when I was in school. I went full-time and worked work-study. I struggled to raise my GPA after it had been so embarrassingly low. I took more classes at the business college, really intrigued by marketing and economics. But nothing was as stimulating and challenging for me as accounting. I could see myself graduating and I was determined to achieve. I said I didn't come all this way to fail. I had to manage my student loan refunds enough to afford my rent and car payments for the semester. I only resorted to calling home after I had exhausted all other avenues to obtain money. Usually, I called on my mother, Auntie Mimi or Moochie (my older brother's father) for money because they always came through for me, but I never asked for more than sixty dollars at one time. I knew my family was also struggling to make it, so I was grateful for any help I was given. My Auntie Bettye gave me a calling card so I could phone the family. Back in those days, we relied on public phones or the dorm room phone which wouldn't dial long distance without a calling card. I always tried to be grateful for any assistance.

I attended my prenatal care doctor appointments regularly throughout the semester. By the time I was four months in April 1998, my stomach had really rounded out—so much so that the nurse at the clinic suggested I get an ultrasound because I was bigger than expected for four months.

At this time, I had a roommate we called Shay, who was my friend from Bunkie, Louisiana and a year older than myself. One of my neighbors at the apartment complex where Shay and I lived introduced himself to us. I had seen Pac around the college of business too. He was from New York and had a confident swag about him. He was also funny and knew I loved to laugh. He told me so many stories about his life, his women, whatever was going on with him. Interestingly, he didn't like Mister because he felt like I deserved better. He saw how hard I was working but didn't see Mister doing anything but kicking it and using my car to do so. Mister didn't like Pac either because he thought Pac was trying to get with me, which wasn't at all true.

Through Pac, I met Zell, also from Chicago, Red from Shreveport, his wife Shon, and other cool people I still know and love to this day. Pac would constantly put me on to jobs and hustle to help make extra money, nothing that would use my body, so I was down. We argued about the top rappers as I did with most guys. What I loved most about Pac is that he saw me as himself, respected my ambition, and never crossed the line with our friendship. He talked about a lot of stuff but had a good heart. I felt safe around him—and that was not easy for me to do. When the semester ended in May, I went to the local hospital in Monroe, Louisiana, about thirty miles from Grambling. This was a "free" hospital, Monroe Clinic, and they treated patients as such. I waited for hours to be seen. Finally, when a resident came in and read my chart, she said she wasn't good at doing ultrasounds, but she would do one on me anyway. The results indicated my baby was fine in size, nothing to worry about. I was happy to hear that because I had planned to go home to Chicago that summer to work. I still had a job at Zonta International downtown, and Lord knows I needed the money. I planned to drive twelve hours from Louisiana to Chicago by myself—five months pregnant—and stay at my mother's house for the summer. I checked the oil, filled the gas tank, and packed to go. I left at 5 a.m., aiming to arrive at my mother's house by 5 p.m. As I drove, I sang to my belly. *The Miseducation of Lauryn Hill* played on repeat in my car's CD player. I was planning to name my son Zion after the Lauryn Hill song of the same name. I only stopped for gas, not even to eat. I drove from Grambling, Louisiana to Chicago, Illinois via Interstate 20, 55, and 57. Louisiana, Mississippi, Arkansas, Missouri sped by, just so I could get see the "Welcome to Illinois" sign. Chicago, only 340 miles away.

MAKING FAITH MOVES

When I began my own family, I learned from the family who raised me what works and what doesn't work for me. I learned that I thrive in peace and receive love through words of affirmation. As a result of growing up the way I did, I didn't want to be involved in a relationship that included any form of physical domestic violence—if I could help it, of course. Once I became a mother, my rule was not to violently argue or fight with my partner in our house with our children. We could go outside somewhere, take a walk or a ride, and talk, but I did not want my children to be involved in grown people's problems. Unfortunately, what you want versus what you get can be two different issues. The final argument Mister and I had in 2007 got loud and very disrespectful. I allowed myself to go as low as he went knowing my babies were in the house sleeping. I felt so bad that I addressed it as soon as they woke up in the morning. I apologized for yelling and cussing and explained as best I could to them at their young ages. Disagreeing with someone doesn't mean you have to be disrespectful to make your point especially for someone you love.

Make people see you and love you at your worth and never settle for less than what you deserve. I had to be patient with myself, my growth and self-discovery. I am a giver by nature; however, I had to set boundaries on who to be a giver to so I wouldn't continue to be taken advantage of.

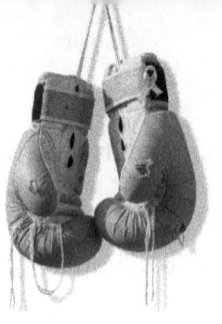

CHAPTER 3

Amiri Baraka:
"HOPE IS DELICATE SUFFERING."

Data from the Centers for Disease Control and Prevention (CDC) from 2018 show that Black women are two to three times more likely to die from pregnancy-related complications than white women, with most of the maternal deaths being preventable. This heightened risk spans all income and education levels. According to the study from the National Bureau of Economic Research, the wealthiest Black woman in California is at a higher risk of maternal mortality than the least wealthy white woman.

Black birthing women are also more likely to experience life-threatening conditions like preeclampsia, postpartum hemorrhage, and blood clots, as well as increased incidence of other pregnancy-related complications like preterm birth and low birth weight. Amid a national reckoning with the systemic racism underpinning American society and healthcare, advocates are pushing forward solutions from multiple angles, including reforming policy, health systems and medical education, and bolstering community-based organizations that advocate for better care and resources for Black moms. The United States is one of only 13 countries in the world where more women die in childbirth today than they did 25 years ago, and African American women are three to four times more likely to die than whites. A black woman with an advanced degree, is likelier to lose her baby than a white woman with an eighth-grade education. Compounding the tragedy, stereotypes with roots in slavery have endured to the present—notably the idea that Black people do not feel pain in the same way whites do, a notion that was used to justify not properly giving black women proper pain medicine.

I read in history books that enslaved women were forced to have children with the enticement of getting out of slavery. If they birthed a certain number of children, they could receive their freedom papers. Slave breeding, a prevalent practice in the slave states, ensured that slave owners would increase their wealth by systematically forcing women slaves to have children. Slave masters raped enslaved women and impregnated them. They also coerced sexual relations between enslaved men and women or girls ending in pregnancies due to forced inbreeding with fellow slaves with the goal of producing a new generation of stronger slaves. In this way, slave owners could increase the number of slaves without having to purchase new stock and to fill labor shortages caused by the eventual abolition of the Atlantic slave trade.

JAY-Z: "I CAN'T TAKE NO THREATS; I GOT A SET OF TWINS"

I began receiving my prenatal care in Chicago after applying for Medicaid, the public assistance for low- or no-income individuals. At one of my appointments, the nurse repeated from the resident in Louisiana had told me: My stomach was bigger than it should be for five months. She sent me to Trinity Hospital to receive an ultrasound. My father and Uncle Boobie went with me to my appointment on June 9th. I remember the date vividly because it was my brother Lonzo's birthday and ten days before mine. When one is on Medicaid, unfortunately, treatment tends to be shit. Regardless of having an appointment, you must wait and wait. By the time they called me for the ultrasound, I was hungry and frustrated. The technician explained the process before she began. As she started, another nurse knocked softly before entering to ask what the technician wanted for lunch because they were ordering. The technician said she was not sure because she would be busy for a while because it was "multiples." The nurse left, and the technician turned to me and said:

Did you hear me? You're having multiples.

"*What do you mean multiples? Can you quantify that for me?*"

"*You are having twins.*"

Long pause, heavy blinking and thinking, before I asked:

"*Can you tell the sex?*"

"*I can see one is a boy and since they are identical twins, they are in the same bag, you're having boys. Congratulations! Do you have any questions for me?*"

As I lay there staring at the ceiling, I said:

"No."

But I had questions for the Lord.

I had set my mind to prepare myself for one baby and finish college. Now, I had to be the mother of two babies at once?

When the technician finished, I walked to the lobby where my father and uncle waited. They stood, and my father shouted happily, "Tell me it's a boy." I shook my head. "No....*two boys*." My father and uncle were so happy I was having twin boys; they were ready to drink to celebrate. On my end, I was in shock. I couldn't wait to call Mister and let him know. When I got to my mom's house, I called him in Louisiana. We didn't have cell phones back then, so I had to try him at different places. I found him at his auntie's house. Mister knew I was having an ultrasound and was waiting for the results. When I told him "Identical twin boys," he dropped the phone. I kept calling his name until he returned and yelled the news to his aunt and cousins.

His family excitedly said we needed to get married—a point which I ignored. I may not have avoided children because I was careless about birth control, but nobody was rushing me to marriage. I had even said at different times that I never wanted to get married. I had a fear of commitment and needed complete control over my life. I knew my control issues, and I put my "all" into it, just like my father used to teach me. "*Don't just do stuff. If you gonna do it, do it 100%!*" Mister's family was from the South and didn't believe in having children without being married. My parents from Chicago may have wanted me to be married before I had children, but they felt at least I was out of the house and made it to college before getting pregnant. All three of my mother's children were having babies in 1998. My sister Jeanette had her second son, and my brother Lonzo's girlfriend was pregnant with their first child while he was serving in the Marines. And then there was me.

I kept working as usual after learning the news of my twin boys. I caught the bus and walked every day from the bus stop. To get to work from my mother's house, I walked from 80th & Colfax to 79th Street for the bus to Jeffrey Boulevard, then caught the #14 Jeffrey bus downtown and walked two blocks to Zonta. As a receptionist, I didn't have to walk; I just sat happily at the front door. After work, I did the routine in reverse. Yes, I had a car by now, but parking in downtown Chicago was expensive. About a week after finding out I was carrying twin boys, and the day after my 22nd birthday, labor pains began. I called my father to go to the hospital with me—I didn't want to wake my mother and stepfather. We arrived at the University of Chicago hospital, where in fact I was born. We attempted to check in at the front desk, but the desk attendant had to ask a ton of questions before getting me a room.

"Have you ever been a patient here?"

"No."

She looked at her computer and said, "It shows you have been here before. According to your name and birthdate you were here on June 19, 1976."

"Fine. I was born here!"

I looked at my father, asking with my eyes, can you believe this? And he chuckled as the pain in my lower back annoyed the heck out of me.

Once I was checked in, a triage nurse checked my vitals, and a doctor checked my cervix and did an ultrasound to examine the babies. They were doing well. It turns out I was only 25 weeks pregnant, way too early to give birth. They said I should have been on bedrest from my fourth month. I informed them I didn't even know I was carrying twins until recently. They were able to get my contractions to stop and sent me home with strict bedrest orders. I dropped my father off at his home and went back to my mother and updated her. My mother scolded me a little when she said to wake them up next time and they would take me to the hospital. The very next night, I began experiencing terrible back pains. I tried lying on the floor and that relief did not last long. I knocked on my mother's bedroom door and announced I wanted to go back to the hospital. My mother and stepdad Larry dressed and met me in the garage. Although Larry took us to the hospital quickly, he was also having severe back pain. My poor Mama had to deal with two suffering people. This time the front desk attendant moved me into triage more quickly. The doctor explained that I was in active labor, and he hoped he could stop the contractions so I could carry out the rest of my pregnancy. Twenty-five weeks was too early, he said: The babies' organs were not developed enough. He said bluntly:

> "If you have these twin boys right now, they will likely not survive."

> "Are you saying I can lose both my babies?"

> "One baby does not have enough blood to exist outside the womb, and if one doesn't make it, his twin will likely not make it either. At this stage, it is hard for one to live without the other. At 25 weeks, the survival rate is 47 to 66 percent. Babies being born at this time will suffer health concerns."

> "What type of health concerns?"

> "If they do make it, their lungs are not developed, their brain is not fully developed, and so on.-Your babies will still be too little to breathe on their own. Babies born at 26 weeks may also develop heart problems."

About 20 percent of babies born at 26 weeks may continue their health problems as they age. These could be problems with vision, hearing, learning, understanding, behavior, social skills. It sounded like nearly everything they would need.

As he shared this devastating news that crushed my heart, he turned and left. The nurse tried to soften the blow. She said the doctor was obliged to tell me all those terrible possibilities, but it did not mean any of it would happen. She cautioned me to hold on to my faith. She said:

> "I have watched you here in the hospital and you seem to be a strong young lady with faith. Trust it."

I was stunned that I could go from zero children to two boys and now possibly back to zero. My mother and I sat in my room, quietly holding back our tears.

From that moment on, I kept my faith. I held my head up and changed my outlook. Hebrews 11:6 teaches us that without faith, it is impossible to please God because anyone who comes to Him must believe that he exists and rewards those who earnestly seek him.

I began praying and talking to God to activate my faith for the sake of my twins' lives.

A couple of hours later, my water broke. My mother called the nurse, and they helped me stand. They set three monitors on my huge belly, one for me and one for each baby. They cleaned my bed and helped back in. Although it was 26 weeks, they said, it was time to have my babies.

The pains were intensifying. At one point, I thought I was having a bowel movement and reached for the bedpan. My mother watched me and started laughing—she knew what that urge felt like when it is time to start pushing babies. The nurse rushed in:

> "What are you doing? You can't just push them babies out yet. We are setting up the labor and delivery room for you."

They quickly dressed me to give birth and got me into position. They coached me. I felt so hot inside my body.

"I'm hot!"

"There's no time for ice now. Mom, you've got to push. The babies must come out."

I had no more energy. I was so hot. I closed my eyes.

My father, who came around that time, later told me it was a code blue. They kicked him out and performed an emergency C-section to extract the babies.

My doctors told me I had no oxygen going to my lungs and I had passed out. A lack of oxygen reaching the lungs, known as hypoxia, can lead to various health problems. It can be caused by conditions that interfere with breathing, such as COPD, asthma, or pneumonia, or by factors like anemia or heart problems. Symptoms include shortness of breath, confusion, and a bluish tint to the skin. Severe hypoxia can be life-threatening and requires immediate medical attention. The human brain can withstand a limited time without oxygen before damage occurs. While survival is possible for a few minutes, irreversible brain damage can occur after 4 minutes, and death can follow within another 2 minutes. Hypoxia, the lack of oxygen, can lead to cell death and damage, with the severity increasing with duration.

When I awoke, I was surrounded: my parents, stepparents, Grandma Janet, Granddaddy, Cousin Karen, aunties and uncles. All I could ask was:

"Did my babies make it all right?"

Yes, everyone nodded. They made it. I went back to sleep.

I woke up in another room, with a nurse checking my vitals. The nurse confirmed the babies were in the neonatal intensive care unit (NICU) and they would take me down to see them after my doctor made his rounds. I went for an MRI and CT scan to confirm why I passed out in labor. My mother told me she heard they wanted to do an Xray to make sure they didn't leave any instruments inside me during the emergency C-section. An emergency C-section is a cesarean delivery performed quickly when there's an immediate concern for the health of the mother and/or baby. It's a form of surgical delivery, where the baby is delivered through an incision in the abdomen and uterus, rather than vaginally. The goal is to deliver the baby within 30 minutes of the decision for the emergency C-section. I had eighteen staples running vertically on my belly right under my navel.

One staff member sat me in a wheelchair after the doctor did his rounds. They took me down to the NICU while explaining the rules, the visiting hours, and the current condition of my twins. There were seven sets of twins in the NICU. When they wheeled me over to see them, my eyes lit up. They were here, finally outside of my belly where they lived for 6 months. They had beautiful shining eyes. They were so tiny. Their skin was translucent. I could see their ribs. Their lungs were not yet developed, and they made no sounds.

Ai explains, babies born at 26 weeks are considered extremely premature, but advancements in medical care have significantly improved their survival rates. While survival is possible, these babies often face many issues with their long-Term health including difficulties with vision, hearing, learning, behavior, or social skills. Babies born at 26 weeks often require specialized medical care in the NICU, including respiratory support, temperature regulation, and nutritional support. One of the complications one of my twins experienced was Intraventricular Hemorrhage (IVH) which is bleeding in the brain. So, I knew we had a long road ahead to get them what they needed to be healthy.

They were beautiful. They were mine. I was in love like I had never experienced in my life. My baby boys were born June 28, 1998.

Baby boy #1, born at 11:11 a.m., weighing 2 pounds, 3 ounces.

Baby boy #2, born at 11:13 a.m., weighing 1, pound 10 ounces.

One of the first thoughts when I saw them was the song by Frankie Valli—but the Lauryn Hill version:

> "You're just too good to be true,
> can't take my eyes off of you,
> you'd be like heaven to touch,
> I wanna hold you so much,
> at long last, love has arrived
> and I thank God I'm alive,
> you're just too good to be true,
> can't take my eyes off of you."

I love you babies!

I sang this to them every day at each visit. I couldn't touch them yet because it was not safe. They were hooked up to so many machines monitoring their heart rate and other vitals. I watched those monitors beep for hours each day, praying my babies would make it out of the NICU. I prayed over them and for their doctors and nurses. I had so many intimate conversations with God during this time. I begged God to let my babies make it out of the NICU. Everyone I knew was praying for my twins. I constantly felt guilty that they were born early, as if I had not protected them. I felt solely responsible for them because they were in my belly. It crushed me. Every day when I left the hospital, I cried because I had to leave them behind. It was like leaving my heart. I internalized this trauma too.

Mister came to Chicago via Greyhound bus from Louisiana to meet our twins two weeks after they were born. I walked around all that summer until they were released as if I was okay, but the Lord knew I was a mess inside. I didn't express my sadness to anyone but God. Visiting hours were from 7 a.m. until 7 p.m. when the nurse switched shifts. We stayed at the hospital, and if a day came when I couldn't go, I felt so bad about leaving them alone. My friends and family gave us a baby shower at my mom's house. My sisters Shantea and Maxine prepared the food and got me an adorable cake in the shape of a bassinet. It was so nice to be smiling even though my babies were still in the NICU. I couldn't wait to get back to them and see their progress and tell them all about their shower, even though they wouldn't really understand. I received baby books and started filling in our family information, including their first footprints.

My faith was strengthening along this journey. I prayed constantly and grew closer to God as I carried my babies. I felt like God was trusting me to bring forth life, and I would not take this responsibility for granted. I was careful about what I ate and drank. I recall my doctor telling me caffeine is not good to drink while pregnant, so I stopped drinking pop and never drank coffee. I dreamed about what I wanted to be as a mother, my vision of being a parent. What would be my legacy? What would I want my children to say about me when I passed? I began talking to God about these concerns. I knew I wanted to protect my children in every way that I never felt protected after I had been sexually abused.

I prayed to be a good mother and asked God for strength, patience, courage, and wisdom. I knew it was up to me to keep them safe, and I vowed to do that until my last breath.

In the NICU they were hooked on the ventilator. A ventilator is a breathing machine used to support premature babies who have difficulty breathing on their own, often due to lung immaturity. It delivers warmed and humidified air to the baby's lungs, essentially breathing for them while their lungs develop or recover. Premature infants, especially those born before 32 weeks, may need respiratory support, including ventilation. Ventilation can trigger inflammation in the brain, increasing the risk of brain injury.

My baby boy #2, whom Mister named Deon, was my 1 pound, 10-ounce preemie—the one doctors said would not make it. He was trying to pull the ventilator out his mouth and nose, so the nurses put a sock on his tiny hands. He also kept trying to take off the sock, so they had to tape the sock around his wrist to stop him from unplugging the ventilator. I smiled to think he was born with such determination to do this his way. I knew then he was resilient and a fighter. Deon was very determined and strong-willed. He was beautiful with his slanted eyes that shimmered every time he looked at you and his smile was priceless with his dimple on his left cheek.

My baby boy #1, whom Mister named Neon, was slightly bigger than Deon. He liked being held and cuddled. Most visits his NICU nurses would be holding him in their arms until we came to visit. He had a deep dimple in his right cheek. Neon was so loving and led with his heart. Neon was handsome with his chubby cheeks and beautiful smile. Neon, like his brother, was resilient and a fighter.

Both boys were perfect to me in their own ways. They made me a better person.

The nurses taught us that preemie babies respond better to skin-on-skin contact—what they called it kangaroo care. Mister held both boys to his bare chest. This helped our babies, and they grew stronger. This practice offers numerous benefits for both the baby and the parent, including improved stability, better temperature regulation, and reduced stress for both. I breast fed them by pumping and storing the milk in bottles for their consumption. They both had to be given blood because they didn't have enough. After this, I chose to become a blood donor every chance I had to give back for what others had graciously given to my babies.

My baby boys were released from the NICU after two and a half months. My first miracles. I will forever be grateful for their lives and fight to survive. They taught me what faith looks like in action.

Becoming a mother was a blessing. As a mother, I realize now that I learned just as much as I taught. I learned patience, unconditional love, humility, and the power of prayer. My stepfather told me God blessed me with two boys at one time because He knew I could handle it. I received that statement and set a vision for myself as a parent to always put them first after God, to be honest with them, to support and love them and discipline them as needed. I talked to God often and asked for help in raising my twins. I planned on teaching them who God is and how to pray. Having boys restored my view of men because I knew their lives mattered, had purpose, and were mine to love unconditionally. My legacy began with them. God showed me through their precious fragile lives how much faith mattered. He showed me how if I used my faith to pray and believe in Him, only good will happen.

MAKING FAITH MOVES

Becoming a mother changed me for the better. I tapped into a place in my heart that had turned cold, especially towards males. My faith in God grew exponentially when I became a mother especially after praying, they survive and watching them fight to be here. I realized if God could get me through this, he could get me through anything.

It was God's will for them to be here; they served a purpose higher than me. My faith was born with their birth. God became my hope and a solid foundation that I would raise my family upon. I knew I wanted to be a parent who showed them more than I told them, so they could see. I didn't believe in the command: *Do as I say, not as I do*. For that reason and so many more, I didn't drink or buy alcohol, and it never appeared in our home until I was 35 years old. I wanted to give my boys the best of everything, including myself as a present parent. I knew they needed me, and I needed them so much. I took them to church wherever we lived because I knew I couldn't raise them without God.

Personally, I was in the bargaining stages of trauma where I realized something happened to me, but I couldn't process it...yet. The result of childhood trauma is a mind that can't be present. It's a constant hypervigilance around who will betray you, abandon you, or what crisis is coming that you can't control. I had to find peace in the presence of God even when going through a storm.

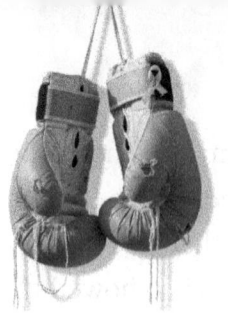

CHAPTER 4

Maya Angelou: "WHEN SOMEONE SHOWS YOU WHO THEY ARE, BELIEVE THEM THE FIRST TIME."

I jumped out the bed from my nightmare, embarrassed that I wet myself as a grown woman and the mother of identical twin boys. I was twenty-two years old. I showered, numb and not a tear fell from my eyes, but I was heartbroken and in pain. I had what seemed like a nightmare off and on, but now I knew it was not a nightmare but my reality.

I had been molested.

Whew. I said it outside my inner thoughts, pushing the words forcefully out of my mouth. When I finished showering, I grabbed a towel hanging over the toilet seat and wrapped it around my body. I told Mister what I recalled of my nightmare as well as everything that had happened to me as a little girl. I didn't share who was involved, but just the events that I remembered. I let it out but then left the bedroom because I couldn't take Mister's stares or see how his looks made me feel ashamed, dirty, and ugly. It always made me uncomfortable when anyone stared at me too long, as if the person could see in the ugliness that happened to me and was living inside of me. I chose to stay hidden under baggy clothes and not try to fix myself to be attractive. Especially after I was raped at 16, I layered my clothing, mostly wearing an extra pair or two of sweats under my slacks. I was skinny back then, so all my clothes were practically sized 0. Sometimes the clothes under my clothes would have blood stains on them from my menstrual period. I continued this until my father confronted me about wearing these nasty clothes that probably even smelled bad. I was embarrassed but couldn't explain to him why I was layering. In my mind, if I smelled and looked unattractive, then no one would want to abuse me sexually. Unhealed trauma can look like low self-worth, and that was my struggle.

Becoming a mother suddenly surfaced all these feelings and emotions in me. For days after my nightmare, it stayed in my mind. I was walking around like nothing was off, but my thoughts were torturing me. Had I repressed these memories since I was a little girl? I struggled with examining if these visions were real or just a dream—or nightmare. My world had forever changed because not only was I raped at 16, but I also mentally battled my memory of molestation between the ages of five and seven. I called my Great Auntie Mimi and shared it all with her. She helped me through by sharing stories of her own sad experiences growing up. My Auntie and I were now trauma-bonded for life. She always offered advice and told me how proud she was of me. We talked often because she saw me—she got me without me having to explain what I meant. She simply understood my motives and intentions, my words and actions.

My days consisted of living in a small one-bedroom apartment with Mister and our twin baby boys on 67th Jeffery Blvd in Chicago. I was working at a company called Zonta International from 8 a.m. until 5 p.m., Monday through Friday. I found a local home daycare center run by an older Black woman and her husband. The state helped us pay for childcare services and we had Medicaid to cover our health needs. My first car, my blue Pontiac Grand Am, had broken down, and I now had a white Buick Skylark that my stepfather Larry cosigned for me. Now we had a more reliable vehicle to take the boys to the physical therapist, pediatrician, and other specialists to make sure they were getting their preemie health services. One specialist looked over our medical files and said we had a lawsuit against the hospital if we wanted to pursue it because I should not have been in labor for seven days. My body couldn't take the stress and so I passed out. My sons were born too soon with developmental delays, one with a blood spot on his brain. The specialist was willing to help.

At that time, I could not think of anything other than making sure my babies were healthy and getting stronger, and that I could pay the rent, car, and whatever else cropped up. I had 99 problems, and I didn't want to start a lawsuit to give me a hundred. The twins received SSI because they were born under three pounds. We received a monthly check of about $500 each. My father got Mister a job where he worked at Hotel Inter-continental downtown Chicago, working with him in the kitchen on the 3-11 p.m. shift. Mister worked for several months, began calling out, and eventually was fired due to his attendance. While it stressed our relationship, I didn't complain much. Who had time to complain? I had to maintain my employment and pay my bills and tend to the twins. We moved into our apartment around September 1998 and signed a year's lease. My job at Zonta was an okay job, but I longed to finish college.

I was feeling like a failure as a college drop out. I investigated transferring my credits to Chicago State University, but it meant losing a year of credits and hard work that I did at Grambling. I continued feeling depressed that my babies were born too early, as if it were my fault. This was my truth: I was a college dropout with two babies and had no idea how to step back on track towards my goals. What goals? I was still fighting inside my head the memory of being molested and raped. Not knowing how to change this drove me crazy. I felt I had no one because the person I was with made me feel as if it was my fault and for me to figure it all out by myself. I was too embarrassed to tell anyone for fear of being judged for choosing someone that couldn't or wouldn't support me.

The year 1999 came in like all the years before, filled with resolutions and hope for a better year. My twins were coming along nicely, hitting their marks slowly but surely. We still visited the specialists. This year, my cousin Karen graduated from Dunbar High School, and we celebrated her achievement.

June 28—the twin's first birthday! I was so happy that my miracle babies had beaten the odds so early in their initial life. I was in awe of them. They already loved music and dancing. They were developing more of their individual personalities beyond their twin bond. Neon was more laid back and Deon was more aggressive. There was no food they didn't like—in fact, they loved eating and insisted on it every two hours, just as they did when I was carrying them in my belly. Mister did all the cooking in our household since I clearly lacked in that area. The boys spoke to each other in their exclusive twin language and cracked up laughing. They were inseparable. We threw them a big first birthday party at the park across from Hyde Park Career Academy High School.

My sister and her boyfriend had given birth to their second son two days after my twins were born, a healthy, happy baby boy named Savon. So, we merged these first birthdays together. Family and friends gathered with joy. Mister barbecued hamburgers, chicken and hot dogs. Family and friends added to the menu by cooking baked beans, spaghetti and potato salad. All three of the 1-year-olds looked adorable even though they had no idea what was going on. We couldn't afford much entertainment like a clown or other performers, so we danced with them to the songs they liked at the time. It was a blessed day.

MAKING FAITH MOVES

I believed and hoped in the potential of those around me even when I was disappointed or harmed by them. I knew Mister was not who I needed or wanted in a husband, but I stayed in our relationship for our little family we started. We were not building anything together, he lived the life he chose, and I did the same with our boys. I was building a life with them and for them. He showed me who he was by being emotionally unavailable, unsupportive, and the financial abuse I encountered in this relationship. When someone shows you who they are, believe them the first time. Unhealed trauma can look like inner shame, codependency in relationships, fear of what happens next.

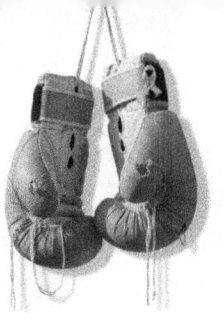

CHAPTER 5

Rakim:
"CONSTANT ELEVATION CAUSES EXPANSION."

My children were on my journey with me from Chicago to Grambling to Cincinnati to Chicago to Fort Wayne, Indiana, and back to the Chicago suburbs. On a quest for stability, I returned with them to Grambling State University to finish college in 1999, graduated July 13, 2001, and took them with me to begin my career in the federal building in Cincinnati, August 13, 2001. My college friend Ayanna asked her mom if I could stay with them for a couple weeks while I was working to find a place to live. My twins went back to my mother's house in Chicago with Mister. I went home on weekends to join them. I worked Monday through Friday in Cincinnati, left the job, searched for reasonably priced apartments (given my low wages).

I was a Grade 5 revenue agent making about 25K a year. Because I couldn't manage much rent, I moved to a low-income neighborhood in Cincinnati. The rent was on a sliding scale according to my income. At that point, Mister brought the twins so we could live together. His brother also moved into our two-bedroom/one bath apartment. His girlfriend, Ayanna, soon joined, and did it become crowded fast.

Since I was the main breadwinner, it was a significant struggle. I had to hold on for another year, when I would get promoted to a Grade 7 agent making 37K. When that happened, I moved from the low-income area to a gated apartment complex with a clubhouse and nice amenities. Mister and I had a hard conversation about our future, including marriage. I shared with him that I simply could not see him as my husband. I could not depend on him for any support for me and the twins.

Truth was, we were leading separate lives. He hung out in the streets with all kinds of strangers. We rarely shared time as a family. More important, he had no idea what kind of woman I was evolving into. I wasn't that naïve college student he met seven years before. He also seldom shows his appreciation for my hard work that kept our family financially stable and the twins healthy. I found them a pediatrician and a dentist wherever we lived. My relationship with God was increasing. I attended bible study each week on my lunch breaks in the federal building and found a church which I and the twins attended every Sunday. I searched for educational experiences for my twins. I brought my sons to museums, the zoo, and local libraries so they could learn to love books and culture.

Mister said he would change. He would show me that he could be all I needed as a husband. He got a second job to supplement his seasonal job. He joined my church and proposed. The pastor of our church gave us premarital counseling. I agreed to marry him because I believed that if we were to remain together, we should be married. Deep down, I knew he had not changed fundamentally. I had to admit as well that I was not in love with him, but I did love him and believed in his potential. He was smart and talented. We were married at our church in Cincinnati by our pastor Culbreath, on the first Sunday of the new year 2003, directly after church service ended. No frills, no thrills. My parents, stepparents, Shantea, and Maxine came down to witness.

While the twins attended daycare on the first floor of the federal building where I worked, they constantly got into trouble for mischief. One day, the daycare called me down because Deon called one of the assistants the N word. The lady's name was Kathy, and she was Caucasian. She proceeded to explain to me that Deon called her the N word even though she was not that color. I asked her what color she had to be to be called the N word. She turned red and said she didn't mean to say that in that way. That day I decided it would be the twins' last day in my building because I could not put out fires and be distracted while trying to learn my job well. I learned our church had a preschool with a few available spots, and it was close to our apartment. The preschool was more diverse, and the location and price fit my budget. The twins stayed there until they graduated from preschool. It seems, as I was to find out later, that Mister was messing around with one of the preschool teachers.

After they graduated, I found a Kindergarten. I taught them the Lord's Prayer that we recited each day before I dropped them off. After the prayer, I played Nas's song "I Know I Can" to inspire and motivate them. We rapped all the lyrics together.

Wanting to stay on track, I learned of a greater career opportunity in another division in Chicago, so I left Cincinnati. I was ready to go home anyway. My mentor and colleague, Elodie, introduced me to Shanita Hicks, a territory manager at that time. Shanita called me into her office and phoned the Chicago territory manager, Jim Daniels, to highlight my educational background and ask about openings in Chicago. They helped me transfer from working in the Tax-exempt Government Entities division in Cincinnati to the Small Business Self-employed division in Chicago. I would go from granting tax exemption to 501(c)(3) and other charitable organizations to examining small businesses and the self-employed. I excelled in my auditing courses at school and found examining income tax returns fascinating. I worked hard to maintain and increase my salary while learning tax law. After all, I was the sole provider and parent of toddler twin boys, as well as a wife, at the tender age of 27.

While living in Chicago, Moochie, the father of my oldest brother rented me an apartment in his building—a two-bedroom/one-bath with a formal dining area and enclosed back porch. Moochie's baby brother, whom we called Uncle Carl, his wife Shavon, and their baby girl Kenyetta lived upstairs, while Moochie lived downstairs. By this time in 2003, I was a Grade 9 agent making 48K a year and upgraded my car from the Buick Skylark to a Pontiac Grand Prix. The building was in the Woodlawn neighborhood where I had grown up, so naturally my twins would attend my former grammar school, Alexander Dumas. Enrolling them in the school where I began my own kindergarten retrieved great memories. I paid my little cousin Kenyetta (who was in high school) to pick them up after school, especially as she lived in our building on the third floor. Even though Mister wasn't working at the time, I did not want him to stay home and watch our twins. I didn't want him to have an excuse not to work, so I simply paid someone to help or found an afterschool program for them until I came home from work. Eventually Mister's sister, niece, and another younger brother came from Louisiana to live with us in Chicago. Even during this crowd, I was the only person working.

The pressure grew every day as I looked at all the bills I needed to cover rent, car notes, car insurance, utilities, groceries, doctor bills, and everything that comes with young children. When I asked Mister about the prospect of a job, even suggesting McDonald's, he turned his nose up and complained about the low pay. He felt too smart to work fast food. I suggested working two jobs then making up for the low-paying wage, like my father used to do. His answer was that he wasn't planning to kill himself working two jobs.

I held my tongue and continued working to take care of my family. I prayed, feeling at the end of my rope. I was exhausted with my home life. I didn't even like to be at home during this time. My life was miserable except for the joy of watching my twins grow. Otherwise, my home was filled with loneliness. Even though I believed in hurting men before they hurt me and cheating back, I was now married. I was in a balancing act, juggling my evolving career, my developing twins, and my sense of inadequacy and entrapment.

Mother's Day, 2005. Mister had stayed out all night. When I got up to get ready for church on that Sunday, I saw my car was gone. I called my friend from around the corner to pick me up so we could visit where Mister usually hung out. As my friend drove by, I spotted my car. I had my key and climbed into my driver's seat and headed home. I readied my boys for church, and we went to fellowship.

My cousin's husband told me he overheard Mister speaking negatively about me, saying that I thought I was better than him because I had a degree or I'm perfect because I attend church. It appeared my success was making him my competition in his mind. He measured himself against what I had achieved and instead of doing the same or better he resolved to hate on me instead and make me his enemy. He wanted to crush my spirit and dimmish my self-esteem. I realized I was literally sleeping with the enemy. He's known me for ten years, and it was hurtful to know how he viewed me after all this time. He resented me and my triumph. I felt it every day. We simply were on opposing teams for a game we could never win.

My friend Maxine purchased a ticket for me to see Joel Osteen. She knew I needed more Jesus. I felt I was fighting for my life. I felt invisible in my own home, overwhelmed and without the tools to communicate how burdened I was.

Each day I woke up to do my job because I was the only mature adult in my house. I was in a challenging career as an accountant in a white male-dominated field. Even here, I had to prove my worth to colleagues who saw me as less than my counterparts. My age and my knowledge were constantly being questioned for me to prove my knowledge, and technical skills were adequate for the work I was to perform. After a full day of work, I returned home and spent time with the boys. Fortunately, mister at least cooked and (most times) cleaned. But in terms of communication about my day, my goals, my life, I was isolated and simply going through the motions of daily living. He had not worked for at least two years at this point, and I felt the weight of it all and it was breaking me.

I enrolled my boys in a program at our church, Apostolic Church of God, called Young Brothers in Christ. Every Saturday morning, they would be with the men of the church and other boys their age. The program leaders were all black men in leadership positions at our church and held leadership roles in their careers. They volunteered their time and resources to teach the boys how to be disciplined, played sports with them, mentored them, and shared their experiences of being Black men. One weekend every summer, the boys went with the program on a camping trip. I sorely needed this time to myself and appreciated this program so much. My cousin Charles stepped up and helped me by picking them up from school until I got off work. My cousin Dwyane helped run my errands. I didn't hang with my sisters Shantea and Maxine often during this time because my marriage was so miserable that I didn't want to transfer that energy to them. When my energy is off, I prefer being alone—unless someone can identify with my situation.

My cousin Tee often picked me up to meet at a club just because I just needed to get out of the house. I also met Tee's friend, Tanya, who I visited regularly. Tanya was hardworking, funny, down-to-earth, loved reading and cool. We all went out one night, and I met him—I'll call him Kelly. When Kelly came over, we talked and laughed at people in the club getting drunk and foolish. Since I didn't drink then, it was all funny to me, just being a grown-up with other grown-ups having a good time. I was overwhelmed committing to work, home, babies, bills, practically ever since I was a teenager in college. I felt walls closing in on me, I felt a lack of love and respect in my home. I knew Mister was cheating and thought I didn't know because I said nothing. Instead, I chose to hang out whenever I could, and I bumped into Kelly often. He showed interest in me and in what I wanted out of life. It was refreshing! He seemed impressed by my career journey.

When I mentioned I had started going to therapy, he asked about my sessions and shared his own issues. We bonded on being in relationships that constricted us because of our children, even though he wasn't married. We walked on the beach just to talk. We shared goals, dreams, and secrets. We talked about affairs I couldn't share with anyone else. He listened to my feelings and allowed me to let down my walls a little bit. I fell in love with him. I shared with Kelly the letter I wrote to my father while in therapy, revealing some childhood trauma that my father didn't know. We both held the capacity for one another to be vulnerable and wanting to fall in love. We developed love for each other at a time we both sought refuge. My connection with Kelly reminded me of a guy I dated in college when Mister I broke up briefly, we will call him Brick City. I could—and did—talk to him for hours.

I had begun an emotional affair that escalated into a physical one later. I was embarrassed at being adulterous. I committed a sin that I was mortified and ashamed of, I didn't recognize myself. I felt like a total failure. However, I also experienced a sense of recognition, affection, and appreciation that had been absent in my relationship at home with Mister. I had been yearning for genuine love, fully aware that such an experience was possible. I was determined to try to live a sin free life by being married and no longer fornicating. I was trying to be a perfect wife and perfect mother and neglected myself for my children's happiness, but I was miserable, found myself being a sinner and felt the weight of that. I felt guilty. This was not the fairy tale *Cosby Show* that I wanted to live. I was not Claire Huxtable, but to be fair, I was certainly not married to Cliff Huxtable either. The weight of being the sole provider of our household and helping his siblings by allowing them to live with us through the years was heavy. I was the only person that worked constantly and consistently. I paid rent, car note, car insurance, utilities, groceries, gas in the car, clothes, shoes, medical insurance, dental insurance, life insurance, you name it, I paid it. I thought I could help everyone achieve the success that I was building for myself. Too many people depended on me, and I felt helpless and lonely. I was unappreciated and taken for granted.

I had to face my demons and do soul searching. My relationship with Mister had distanced me from my own character, and I hated that for myself. We were on a vicious toxic cycle. He would hurt me, but instead of arguing about it, I wanted to pay him back for the pain he caused me. Mister confronted me about my affair. He found my hotel bill from my business trip to Dallas that listed all the numbers

I called. I couldn't lie, so I admitted what happened. I told him when it began, where I met Kelly, and what feelings I had for him. I shared my unhappiness. Mister said I had not done anything for him, so he did not understand why I felt overwhelmed. He said, I would have had all those bills anyway, whether we were together. He wanted me to give him more or buy him things which I flat out refused. I was disgusted. I was done. I purchased him a one-way Greyhound bus ticket to Cincinnati to stay with his brother. We parted ways while his sister, niece, and younger brother still lived with us.-

Eventually, I also ended it with Kelly. I knew it was wrong to start a relationship before ending my marriage. I told him I couldn't continue what we had until my divorce was finalized, and he understood but said he would always be there for me. I felt his pain in my decision. It gave me Deja-vu when I broke up with Brick City in college to put my family back together. This time, I was not repairing my family. I was choosing my happiness. I left Mister for myself, my peace, my sanity, and my promise of a love I wanted and deserved. Through that time, I got stronger and remembered who I was as a woman with needs that exceeded the bedroom. I had to find my voice and stand up for what I wanted. Never again would I settle for less. So began my transition to being a single mother, officially.

As a single mother, I wanted to ensure my sons had all that their friends with two parents had—from their own bedrooms with TVs and computers to family vacations to a different state each year. I feared for their safety growing up in this world as a black man. I worried about them every time they were away from me. I worked hard to get them out of the neighborhood where I grew up in Chicago that was no longer family friendly. My mother became my model because I saw what she had done when she and my father divorced. My mother still raised us in our own place by herself. I witnessed my mother purchasing her first house as a single mother. I had plans for home ownership too and saw all its benefits. It was a challenge to learn how my credit score could impact my chances of becoming a homeowner. My credit score had been damaged from the credit cards I had used while I was in college buying books and supplies. I attended my first-time buyer classes to educate myself on the home-buying process. I set up a plan to achieve this goal by myself. After one too many car break-ins, mice in my apartment, ridiculously light and gas bills, gunshots, random acts of violence, I knew I had to move. I gave up the apartment and moved to Fort Wayne, Indiana, because I could transfer my office there. It also was still close to Chicago and more affordable for my goal of homeownership. I stayed with the boys at my mother's house until I had enough money to move.

Christmas 2005 was spent in Charlotte, North Carolina, at my maternal grandparents' home with my twins, my mother, and Aunt Bettye. I drove us all down south to North Carolina like my Grandfather Clarence used to do when we were children. On our way back to Chicago, I dropped the twins off with their father and his family in Cincinnati—all his siblings had come together by now. This was the first time I had been without my twins for a week and a half. I enjoyed the taste of freedom, but being by myself became boring after two days. I couldn't call on Kelly to hang out with me since I wanted to wait until my divorce was processed. I still craved attention from the opposite sex. I admit I needed validation from men, words of affirmation and attention to make me feel better. I met a guy while I was running errands at Taco Bell on 79th Stony Island. We talked on the phone a few times before setting up a date to hang out with him at my mom's house. Whenever I met guys now, I always made it clear that I was not interested in having sex, just so they would remove that possibility from their minds.

I was honest about my current situation of being separated and working towards a divorce.

I was date-raped at my mom's house January 2006. The guy I met came over as we planned and we watched TV, talked, and shared some laughs before he decided to move to the sofa where I was sitting to get closer to me. I reminded him of my no-sex rule, to which he agreed. As time passed, he moved closer, even sharing the couch now. I felt nervous but didn't show it. I was aware of how I was alone in the house with a man I didn't know. My intentions were pure, but he was not. He raped me. I lay there not moving, frozen, until he got off me. I was again the little girl being molested and the 16-year-old being raped. I was hurt beyond pain. I tried to trust the male species again, yet again I was abused. I don't recall what was said before he left. I locked the door, ran upstairs, and took a long shower, my tears mixing with the water. I became broken again. I didn't tell anyone. I felt embarrassed and ashamed.

If I shared this with anyone, they would judge me for letting him in my house while I was alone. I feared no one would believe me or judge me so I didn't share this with anyone but God. I shook it off as though nothing had happened. It is unfair that a woman cannot just hang out with a man without suffering abuse. I even heard that of a question asking women if they felt safer in a room by themselves with a man or a bear. Most responded bear. I've heard too many stories like mine, unfortunately. The sad part was that however far I had come, my mental state had become more messed up now than even before.

Two days later, I drove to Cincinnati to collect my twins from their visit with Mister and his family. It was a cool visit, and it was clear that he was moving on as I was from our relationship. However, we shared an intimate moment because it was familiar for both of us. Sex was my vice, as I've said, and I could detach myself from the act. My vagina was still sore from being raped two days ago, however, because he was familiar to me and I needed something that I felt I could control, I allowed it. This time it wasn't taken from me. It was like putting a band aid on an open wound. If there was one thing Mister and I knew how to do well, it was sex. But this time, I knew there was nothing left there for us. It did not feel the same anymore. It didn't fix the pain of being sexually assaulted so I internalized my agony again. Afterwards, I lay in bed thinking, I had to follow up on my divorce once and for all, it was time. I was so scarred on the inside.

In April 2006, I found out I was pregnant. My emotions were scattered everywhere. I had no plans and dreaded having another baby in this relationship. I made an appointment to have an abortion, but I couldn't do it. I had experienced an abortion before, and it tore me up emotionally. I attended service at Apostolic Church of God where Bishop Arthur M. Brazier was preaching and teaching about how in the days of the bible, they marched to the city of Zion to pray. His message on that Sunday was what I needed to hear. I knew I could not proceed with aborting this baby I was carrying. I cried out in emotional pain and anguish, realizing that I would carry this baby at such a tumultuous time in my life. I was grieving over the death of my marriage and the loss of Mister as a friend.

God knew. He came to me and told me this baby was my blessing, no matter what. I trusted God and needed to get my mind together for the sake of this pregnancy and thereafter.

I endured so many criticisms, questions, and comments about my baby and his father. I didn't fold under pressure or noise. I trust God, even though it does not always look that way. I never really cared what people said or thought of me mainly because of my relationship with God. However, in this season, I heard it all—even from people I never expected would question my character. I was aware of people who were secretly competing with me to see if I would fall or fail. More than ever, I had to trust God. It was a dark, lonely, and hurtful time filled with unkind comments about me and my baby, but I knew God would use this test as my testimony. Obedience is greater than sacrifice, and as I carried this baby, I was obeying God. I fell in love with carrying this child in my belly as I had when I carried his brothers. Nothing else mattered to me but keeping my baby safe and delivering a healthy child. I truly enjoyed feeling the baby grow in my body.

Once we moved to Fort Wayne in August of 2006, I was a little more than six months pregnant and my cousin Stafford and his wife, Tracey, let us stay with them while I looked for an apartment. My plan was to rent for one year, then buy my house. I found a nice affordable two-bedroom/two-bath apartment. I researched schools and pediatricians for my twins. It wasn't hard to transfer my job from Chicago to Fort Wayne, just as I had done from Cincinnati to Chicago—one perk of working for the government. My soon-to-be ex-husband moved from Cincinnati to Fort Wayne to be with us. We were still legally married, even though the connection was gone, as his actions continued to demonstrate. I transferred my prenatal care to an obstetrician/gynecologist in Fort Wayne. I learned I was carrying a baby boy and planned carefully for his birth with my doctor.

On October 24, 2006, at 2 p.m., I gave birth to Zion, a beautiful healthy baby boy born by a scheduled C-section. I was fully awake when they pulled him out of my belly. It was one of my happiest days to see a healthy baby being born from my body. Despite the ugliness that had happened to me, my beautiful, beautiful Zion was indeed my blessing, just as God said he would be. His eyes met mine and connected with love. He was larger than both of my twins together, and his skin was so red. I hadn't witnessed my twins' birth, so this was indeed a glorious blessing. I named him Zion, although Mister wanted me to name him Keon. I wanted to give him my maiden name Knox, but Mister declined since we were still legally married. The family loved my new addition to my family. He was a welcome blessing to our family. I had given birth to three of the most handsome and happiest boys. I was ecstatic. Of course I sang Lauryn Hill's song, to Zion to my baby boy just as I had with his brothers.

> "Unsure of what the balance held, I touched my belly overwhelmed, by what I had been chosen to perform. But then an angel came one day, told me to kneel and pray, for unto me a man-child would be born. Woe this crazy circumstance. I knew his life deserved a chance, but everybody told me to be smart, "Look at your career, " they said, "Lauryn, baby use your head". But instead, I chose to use my heart. Now the joy of my world, Is in Zion! Now the joy of my world, Is in Zion!"

Mister found a job working nights once I went back to work because he didn't want anyone to watch Zion. We were still leading separate lives, and I had no idea where he went, who he hung up with, or how he spent his time away from our family. He chose to hang out with one of my younger cousins instead of my cousin that was more our age.

One day, Mister told me he had found a babysitter for Zion during the day while he rested before going to work at night. I already knew this must be someone he was dating because he never found a school, daycare, or program for our children before, so I waited until he introduced her to me. I could tell she liked him—it was all over her face. I told him my observations later, and of course, he denied it, saying she preferred girls, so she probably liked me instead. I knew better and trusted God to reveal it to me when the time was right. I didn't have to go looking for proof. I knew it just would come.

One pitfall of removing my children from the city to a smaller town with less violence is racism. I was raising Black boys to men, and for them to experience racism hurt my heart. When my twins were in the second grade, their principal called me early in the morning to say she would suspend my son for coming into her office yelling that morning about what had happened on the school bus. I asked logically what happened to him on the school bus. She replied, "*I don't care what happened, I'm concerned with how he entered my office yelling.*" I repeated to her what she said to me, and she continued as if everything was fine. When I hung up, I transcribed our conversation and faxed it to her supervisor, with a copy to the principal, the U.S. Department of Education, Fort Wayne Community Schools administration, and even Judge Greg Mathis. I found out that my son-shine (that's what I call my sons) was upset because for the first time in his young life, a white boy called him a Nigger on the school bus. Immediately, she called me to set up a meeting. Mister and I attended. The principal was physically frustrated and explained how she had been "*more than kind to you people*"—and this instantly ended the meeting for us. We left pissed.

In response to my complaint to the Fort Wayne Community Schools supervisor, the principal had support staff falsely report to Child Protective Services (CPS) that my twins were being abused and neglected. She used CPS as a weapon for payback. CPS instantly removed them from school and placed them in a stranger's home. They claimed a couple of scars on their knees were reasons to remove my children from my home until we had court that week. I hired an attorney to fight this unfounded claim. The same principal who had not cared about what happened to my son on the school bus days earlier now cared about them being abused and neglected. This claim occurred at the end of the school year. It had no basis, and everyone knew it. My boys had been visiting the pediatrician regularly since they were born, and no one had ever voiced any issues or concerns with their well-being. They were rough-playing boys who loved sports and fought each other and others sometimes, so explaining the presence of a scar on their knees was preposterous. Nonetheless, the attorney advised me of his fee if I chose to fight this claim. He suggested letting it play itself out, allowing CPS to visit my home during the year to check they were not abused and/or neglected. Once again, I felt defeated. After that year, I received a letter from CPS closing the case and clearing us.

My sons were seen as criminals as early as the second grade, and when I fought against the system, they punished my family by removing them (temporarily) and weaponizing state-funded programs in a felonious charge. They never apologized or admitted the principal was wrong in her actions. Ultimately, the Fort Wayne Community School system removed that principal from that school the following year and transferred her elsewhere. That was also the last year for my twins at that school. Unfortunately, the racism didn't end there.

I taught my children Black history. I bought books with characters that looked like them to reinforce their identity and affirm them as brilliant, handsome Black boys. In February, during Black History Month, I assigned projects for the entire month, requiring my children to research notable Black and African American historical figures, inventors, writers, artists, athletes, and politicians. I wanted them to learn their history so they could value themselves even more by knowing their rich history in this world. I made everything a learning experience, even when I punished them. I asked them to look up words in the dictionary and write the definitions or read a book about something they struggled with and compose a paper on what they learned.

In August 2007, I closed on my first house that was being specially built. It was 2,200 square feet, four bedrooms/2.5 bathrooms, with an unfinished basement, and I designed every inch of it myself. I accomplished my goal of purchasing my first house at the age of 31. I went by myself to find a real estate agent, got pre-approved, and decided to build a house instead of purchasing a prebuilt home. I decided every inch of what my house would look like and the structures I wanted. I paid my closing cost alone. At this time, I was involved in the CPS case started by Fort Wayne Community Schools but had also just received a promotion at work. I was the only one to see the house until I closed on it and took Mister and my gentlemen to see it. My gentlemen were so excited to see it, they ran throughout the house. I searched the schools in Fort Wayne to find a diverse area before choosing where I would build. The area was nice, centrally located in the town. I was so proud of myself and my accomplishment, even if Mister never told me so.

Since I had just paid a significant amount of money for the house, closing cost, and other expenses, I could not afford much for movers, so I suggested Mister ask Zion's babysitter to use her father's truck to help us move into the house and she obliged. I wanted another chance to see her again and pick up on her vibes. My woman's intuition confirmed what I already knew to be true. I saw it in her face, as she stared and compared herself to me. Interestingly, I began receiving private phone calls to my cellphone and when I answered, no one said anything.

Two days later, this girl screwed up courage to tell me that she had made many attempts to call and play these phone games. I antagonized her enough until she finally found her voice and admitted that Mister was cheating on me with her. She said she was in love with him. I could tell she expected me to be aggressive with her, but I surprised her. I told her good, now he can live with her and her father in their shack. I promptly packed Mister's clothes in the newly constructed house I had built for us, drove them to her father's shack where they were staying, and left them on the front porch. I called our cellphone carrier, informed them that I "lost" the phone he had, and requested that they disconnect that line. I called a locksmith to change the locks on my doors so he could not enter my house. I was finally removing all trace of him and me from this toxic relationship. He lived with the girl and her father, so I had no worries about where he would stay anymore if I left him. I filed for divorce that week, and it was finalized a year after Zion was born. Zion had indeed been my blessing for so many reasons.

MAKING FAITH MOVES

I was in the anger stage of trauma where I accepted something had happened and I was angry about it. In addition to going through trauma, I was grieving the death of my relationship with Mister. The five stages of grief are denial, anger, bargaining, depression, and acceptance. I experienced every stage of grief with Mister. I was demonstrating loyalty by taking care of him and his family members with the hope he would be loyal to me. I wish he had shown that he valued me and our children by working hard and easing my burden a little. But once I accepted who he was instead of who I wanted him to be, I could no longer sustain this relationship. It was killing me. I suffered financial and psychological abuse. I accepted it. Staying with him was misery. Psychological abuse can have a profound impact on someone's mental health. Victims can feel trapped, threatened, humiliated, used, or a combination of all these. Most signs therefore relate to someone's mental state, and changes in behavior: Helplessness. Being unhappy at home did not make me a good parent because I was emotionally checked out. I was annoyed and disappointed in my relationship, so I sought love from another man instead of doing internal work on myself. My tolerance finally ended when I filed for a divorce in February of 2007. I had lost myself but needed to remember who I am and whose I am. I am a child of God, and I knew God did not want any of this for me. Progress comes from shifting your environment and mentality with new information which causes expansion of the mind.

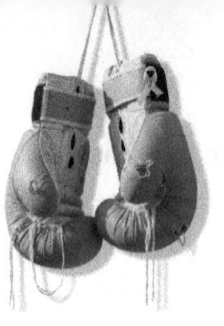

CHAPTER 6

Tupac:
"SO NO MATTER HOW HARD IT GETS, STICK YOUR CHEST OUT, KEEP YA HEAD UP…AND HANDLE IT."

I had Zion's first birthday party at our new home. Since his birthday is so close to Halloween, that was the party theme. I hired a makeup artist to do the children's face painting, we made balloon animals, held dancing contests and games. Immediately after his party, my friends and I had "Lady's Night" at my house. My sister friends travelled from Chicago, Wisconsin, and Rock Island to join the party. We began having ladies' night out once a month, hosted by a different lady each month. Our lady's night out crew usually consisted of myself, Jeanette, Maxine, Woodie, Belinda Nicole, Erica, Shavon, Esha and Ne-Ne. Other women joined depending on who was hosting and what activities we chose.

 We hosted these events from January until October, with October being the grand finale since we knew November and December were busy with our families for the holidays. We traveled with our children sometimes; it was a family affair but mostly a way to remain connected with each other without phones and social media. It was a safe space to connect, discuss, to support, show love and stand in prayer together. We closed out every lady's night out with prayers usually led by Maxine. This was sisterhood. Sisterhood is acceptance. Sisterhood is understanding, compassion and loyalty. Sisterhood means supporting each other without judgement and standing up for one another. We advocate and defend each other, address mistakes privately, and practice honestly even when it involves tough conversations or expressing hurt feelings. Sisterhood is accountability without dire consequences; we give grace as we evolve into our higher selves.

There were so many challenges of raising three sons on my own. Being a young mother to Black male children living in America is hard. The statistics for the sons of single mothers turning into criminals are disturbingly high. I have always heard stories of the man of the house leaving and the woman going down, but I refused to allow that to happen to me. I worked, hustled, budgeted, planned, worked, cried, prayed, won battles, and learned lessons, but I never lost. When I had to go out of town for work, I called on my family to help with my boys. For one trip where I had training in Maryland, my Auntie Bettye came down to Fort Wayne to watch the boys in my house; another time, my Uncle Tony came from Chicago to help me while I had training in California.

I never asked the same person for help more than once because I never wanted to burden any one family member with my responsibilities. When I moved to Cincinnati, my great-grandmother and Auntie Mimi kept the twins for a while because I didn't trust Mister to do it full-time. When I went to California, Mister assured me that he could watch his boys himself at my house, but I let him know Uncle Tony would be there, regardless. I left them with my car, and money for groceries, and anything else they needed. Unfortunately, when Mister tried to help, he kept the money and broke my garage door by "accidently" hitting it with my car—and that cost me $800. Not only was he not helping but he also became a liability. It was a delicate balance with Mister because it was important to have his physical contributions; the boys needed his presence in their lives, and I would never stand in the way of his parenting them, even if he made no other contributions. I did not care to control who he spent time with or what activities the boys engaged in when they were with their father. I simply respected Mister's contribution as a father was different than mine as a mother. I love my boys far more than whatever I might have felt toward their father.

I took the boys on out-of-state trips whenever I could manage. Their first time flying was to attend the high school graduation of my little brother Elijah in Phoenix, Arizona in 2009. The twins were now eleven and Zion was two going on three. I was so anxious about how Zion would act on this flight. To my surprise, he did well, never once embarrassed me by crying on this four-and-a-half-hour flight. One summer, my friend Deborah told me about a children's summer camp in Wisconsin, and the rate seemed reasonable for my twins. Unfortunately, the twins didn't last the two weeks away at camp—they got kicked out for mischief, so my sister Maxine kept them until I arrived the next day to pick them up. My other sister Shantea kept them for a week or two in the summer, and I always appreciated any help I received.

In the summer of 2010, I wanted the boys to connect more with their father's side of the family. Mister's two brothers came to Fort Wayne from Cincinnati to help me drive them down to Monroe, Louisiana. Mister didn't want to go, so his brothers went in his place. I had not made this 12-hour road trip in many years, but I drove all of us down there in July for a month with relatives. The boys hated the hot weather and the bugs that came with it, and they were ready to return after just a week! I drove back down there two weeks later to pick them up because my Uncle Jobe was terminally ill with cancer, and I needed the boys back with me; if I waited too long, I wouldn't be mentally nor emotionally able to drive 12 hours.

In 2011, I trained for two weeks in Nashville, Tennessee, and brought my Son-shines along with me. My twins were now twelve going on thirteen and Zion was four going on five. While I trained during the day, I let the boys sleep in the hotel with their new Nintendo handheld games. My stepsister Ebony came to visit us in Nashville, because she lived in the area. When I had free time me and my boys visited the local attractions in Nashville, and I brought everyone cowboy hats! The following summer, my sons visited my father and stepmother in Phoenix, Arizona for two whole weeks, all three of them flying on their own like big boys. I joined them two weeks later and we flew back home together. We visited museums and local zoos anywhere we travelled. We visited the National Underground Railroad, known as the Freedom Center, in Cincinnati and to the Newport Aquarium in Kentucky. Zion was fascinated by dinosaurs, so we went to the exhibits at the Children's Museum in Indianapolis and Lincoln Park Zoo in Chicago.

I constantly attended meetings with Fort Wayne community schools regarding how my sons were treated in their classes. I met with teachers and administrators to decide on what was best for them and discipline them for every little episode that required it. I went to those meetings with the strength of God and standing on the shoulders of my ancestors. I was usually the only Black person in the room. It never fails to astound me that educators with no experience with Black Americans were running their education. I asked each person in the room to tell me their name, title, and involvement with my children. The way they looked at me and talked about my children was with audacity and contempt. To them, I had nerve to question them and their qualifications. Who did I think I was?

When my twins were in middle school, the school had an issue with all sixth-grade boys fighting in the bathroom. To combat this issue, the school decided that when the next fight occurred, the 12-year-old boys would be locked up for fighting. One of my boys was in the bathroom when a white student entered and pushed him into the bathroom wall. In self-defense, my son punched the boy in the face and broke his glasses. They arrested my son but not the white student and called to inform me afterwards. My 12-year-old son with no prior issues or exposure to the law, the police, or the criminal justice system was taken into custody. I was not allowed to see him that day, and I cried myself to sleep with anger and worry because my son suffers seizures and has a diagnosed learning disability. In the morning, I saw the judge who immediately dismissed the charges and threw out the case. The anxiety I felt because of this injustice caused me to have a small stroke, or TIA. As a single Black mother, I felt the weight of the world on my shoulders. I felt defeated, as if all my efforts were futile. Part of me, though, continued to trust that I was doing what was right, and I believed if I just stayed consistent, I would one day reap what I had sowed.

Here, I had chosen to move my family from Chicago to a better place, only to experience the racism of a small town. By the end of 2011, we moved back closer to Chicago. I fought for them daily in the school system, in the healthcare system, any system that was denying my boys their rights. In the aftermath of all these upheavals, my Son-shines and I started family as well as individual therapy. I know I was raising them in survival mode and in that vein, there really is no room for emotions, its strict discipline. In this state, the brain prioritizes basic safety, immediate problem-solving, and essential needs, often at the expense of complex thinking, long-term planning, or self-care. During survival mode, processing emotions beyond immediate needs is challenging. I realized they needed more support, but I lacked emotional intelligence then. Although I expressed love through words and actions, I couldn't heal the pain caused by their father not being active in their lives anymore. They experienced challenges related to their father's absence, which affected them. They were unable to express their feelings about missing their father's presence in their daily lives as they had before. For their whole lives, I involved them in church, sports, and clubs like Big Brothers, Boys and Girls Club, young brothers in Christ, and 100 Black Men of Chicago. They always had a male role model to teach them how to be men because I knew I could not.

I wanted to find out how the seizures were affecting my sons' brain and determine where they both stood academically. I wanted to make sure they were healthy in every way: physically, mentally, emotionally, and spiritually. I set them up with a psychoneurological assessment through the University of Chicago. I sat in the ER alone whenever my son would have a seizure, and one of my friends, Natasha or Rhonda in Fort Wayne, watched my other two boys. I advocated for him to get the best care, maintained excellent health insurance, took him to specialists, and followed up with every concern about his medicine and how it affected his development. I always prayed for my sons because I knew they would have difficulty maneuvering life without me. They had developmental delays, and Mister was mostly absent from their lives. Even though he was in the same town, he was sporadic in calling and visiting, sometimes six months would pass without a word from him.

My pressure continued to increase. There were just no days off from life. I had to learn how to balance my career to remain competitive for promotions but not allow my career to overshadow my children. I had to balance my parenting, conscious that I was raising boys to men, so I could not coddle them, but I needed them to feel loved and safe. Of course, I was supposed to be the nurturer, but I had to turn into the disciplinarian as well. I had a tough equilibrium to maintain. I had to teach them structure, order, and firmness. Even I changed because of this: Any softness in me turned into aggression. I didn't affirm them as I should have, or I minimized conversations with them to ask how they were feeling with family shifts and many little things that were important. I regret that.

I found a sitter for Zion, which is more local to our neighborhood because it became too much for me to travel around in the mornings dropping off kids in different places. Mrs. Rachel was a blessing.

I stayed in survival mode. Being in a "good neighborhood" had become critical because I knew how easily the streets or peers can manipulate young boys into doing the wrong stuff. I know firsthand how even just a walk to the bus stop can be dangerous. I had to find the best pediatricians, dentists, specialists, barbers, role models, recreational activities, church, and schools. I had to protect their bodies, minds, and spirits. I had to make good money, save, budget, and plan family vacations. I had to make my work schedule compatible with their school schedule, so I saw them off on the school bus and met them back home after school. Thank God for companies that use the alternative work schedule (AWS). Even prior to the COVID-19 lockdown, I was able to work from home any day I chose and split my workday. I would start work at 8:30 a.m. after the twins left on the bus and I dropped Zion at daycare. I left work at 2 p.m. to meet the twins from the bus by 2:30 p.m. and bring them to their afterschool program at the Urban League or Boys and Girls Club, until return to work around 3 p.m. and officially ended at 5:30 or 6. Once I picked them up—if they didn't have more activities, like karate, tutoring, therapy, church rehearsal, basketball or football—we finally went home. The twins would zip through our backyard to Mrs. Rachel's home to pick up Zion.

Once resettled, everyone changed clothes, sat at the table to do homework, while I helped and cooked dinner. We even managed a few bonding hours to find out what was going on at school or if they needed anything before bedtime. They then showered, cleaned the bathroom after themselves, prayed, and went to sleep after a full day! I usually took an hour of total downtime for myself, maybe cleaning up good enough for me to rest. At one point, I hired a cleaning lady to come once a month and do a thorough scrub. All bills belonged to me, and there were no complaints. I knew it was all part of the territory of raising children well. I didn't have a lot of extra time or money to spare, but what I was accumulating was peace.

My children were happy and that's all that mattered to me. Zion literally jumped into my arms whenever I picked him up from daycare. We always ran to each other on sight, and I said, "I love you superstar" and he answered back, "I love you, fat arms!" His teachers were appalled to hear him call me "fat arms," but it didn't bother me one bit because he was obsessed with my arms. He loved to kiss my arms and hang on to them. The twins and I had dance contests on the Wii and rapped songs together. It was me and the boys against the world in some ways, and these little men helped restore my disappointed feelings about the male species.

The young girl Mister cheated with used to harass me with phone calls all hours of the night. She even called CPS to report I had drugs in my house, and an agent came to my brand-new house to investigate before throwing out the claim as unvalidated. I never received one penny of child support for seven years, as our divorce decree was mandated. But I still allowed the boys to see Mister whenever he called or came. I even allowed his girlfriend to pick them up, even though there was a restraining order against her for threats and harassment against me. I knew my sons had a right to have a relationship with their father, despite my feelings towards him. I advocated for their relationship so much that when he wouldn't come around or call for months at a time, I still purchased gifts and wrote Mister's name on them as if those presents came directly from him for his sons. I constantly made excuses for him to them, but I never spoke negatively about him or his girlfriend while my children were around. I learned this from my parents when they split—neither ever spoke badly about the other in front of me. I believed that one day, the boys would find out exactly who their father is in their own time, but not from me. His actions would dictate all they would ever need to know.

I prayed that God would give me strength to not take vengeful actions against him. I asked more of the spirit of God in me to allow God to fight my battles. Through all these issues, I prayed and repeated the scripture: Greater is HE that is in me than he that is in the world. Through it all, I stood tall and responsible in raising my men as it was principally up to me how they viewed the world and—most importantly—how they viewed and treated women. Despite the endless expenses and bills, I paid the price to be the boss of my home with as few complaints as possible. I wanted to give my children the gift of a worry-free, happy, and safe childhood.

I had issues handling microaggressions at work since I was one of a few Black revenue agents in Fort Wayne, working with white men who clearly had never interacted with Black people. My white counterparts would mention in conversations Black stereotypes and ridicule Black celebrities with criminal backgrounds. Interestingly, they never mentioned white celebrities with criminal backgrounds in the news. Indiana and Ohio are not like Illinois (specifically Chicago), and it showed. My colleagues claimed they never heard of my college and asked why I felt the need to attend a Historically Black College and University (HBCU). My colleagues questioned my feelings about the O.J. Simpson murder trial and why Black people were happy with the verdict since two white people were killed. I asked if they had ever heard of Rosewood, Emmett Till, Black Wall Street, or Medgar Evers. No, they said. Some colleagues asked me if they could touch my hair.

If a conversation came up about the transatlantic slave trade, my colleagues would make it a point to inform me that their grandparents or parents also came over to America from a foreign land, had to learn English, had to earn a living, and aimed for the American Dream to create generational wealth. I pointed out the contrasting perspective: My ancestors crossing the Atlantic came not by choice but by coercion, kidnapping, beating. They were lynched for learning how to read, and the generational wealth they could have established with the promise of 40 acres and a mule was not honored. My intelligence was always in question, and I felt I had to teach them about rules of dealing with diversity.

When I entered the field of accounting, I earned my degree to gain a position with a company I could grow with, a company that valued a work-life balance and helped me develop a skillset. I worked to be a provider for my family and earn an honest living. I was no different than the rest of my colleagues, and yet they saw me as totally different.

I don't believe I ever learned how to balance work, parenting, and self-care simply because I never factored in self-care for myself. If I had to "punish" my boys, I would stay in the house, so essentially, I was being punished too. I learned to shift and pivot. When I made mistakes, I accepted my accountability for them. I figured out what I did wrong and regrouped. I was constantly living for the next moment, next event, next appointment, not living in the present because sometimes, yes, the present was painful. My reality was that I was raising three Black boys to be men as a single Black woman. I was entirely responsible for their everyday lives, every article of clothing, every food they ate, what they learned or read, how their health turned for the better or not. Nothing could be taken for granted or lost.

This was particularly difficult as my twins were on the spectrum and Neon had epilepsy. At any given time if he was stressed or had a fever, he could seize, so it was my job to keep him stress-free and prevent attacks. He was having them so frequently at one point, I asked his neurology team about medication I could administer instead of running to the ER each time. I was given Diazepam with the dial already set for his weight; it had to be administered through his rectum. When he was going through a grand mal seizure, so I had to turn him on his belly and insert the dial into his rectum, so the medication went straight into his bloodstream. I prayed constantly that my children would bury me, not the other way around. There was no one in my family who could relate to these exact challenges I was going through. I was so used to being on my own that I never asked for help for fear of being disappointed, as had happened so frequently.

In 2011 due to lack of family support with my children and racism in Indiana, I decided to sell my house that I designed. I requested a work transfer to the Chicago post of duty to move from Fort Wayne, IN. While trying to sell my house, my real estate agent advised me to remove all the family pictures, and black art I had on my walls especially the picture of Obama because a white family will not purchase a house once owned by a black family. Although I was insulted at first, I set aside my feelings to focus on selling my house. I was relocated to the Shiller Park, IL office for work and found a house to rent in Lansing, IL for me and my Sunshine's. My older brother moved in with us in the spring of 2012 with his younger son.

When they were freshmen in high school, I took the twins to a psychoneurological assessment at the University of Chicago Hospital. I wanted to see the effect of the seizures he had on Neon and see Deon's levels were since he didn't want additional assistance in school or for himself. The assessment was an eight-hour battery of tests on intelligence, academics, and social and behavioral aptitudes. I was moved to hear one doctor's observation: that my sons had a good mother and a village that raised them well. The reality was that it was easy for young Black boys to have criminal records by this age. The doctor praised the twin's respectful behavior. However, the disappointing news was that Neon would not be able to obtain a regular high school diploma or achieve good results from higher learning. They suggested teaching him life skills and not much else. They said Deon was more progressive than Neon, but they did not recommend college for him either. It hurt me as a mother that my boys would not be considered "regular."

It hurts when bullies call either of them retarded or slow. I always wanted my children to make their own choices and decide what they wanted in life with no limits. And God knows I know the added complications of making it in the world as Black Americans. Now their hurdle was being special needs in school with a prison pipeline set as early as second grade. This doctor was telling me that both boys, and more so Neon, had limits.

I have always struggled with the idea of perfection. This prognosis was the opposite of perfection. I was devastated but my sons could not see me being distraught. This is another burden to keep inside. I did not know anyone going through the same could help me come up with—if possible—a positive outcome.

The twins struggled through school. By the time they reached high school, some of the antics they exhibited earlier in their academic career were limited. I had them complete my own assignments on how to budget money, how to find an apartment, and how to live on your own. I incorporated this idea into my children's lives after I taught a few financial literacy classes at the Come as You Are Church. I started off teaching them about credit—including keeping their name clean and their credit good. A clean name means honoring your word and staying out of the criminal justice system. I had no issues with Zion's performance in daycare or in school. He was a good student and seemed to love learning.

In their junior year of high school, I was over my twins' failing classes, given all the resources they had available to them. We stayed up late nights reviewing homework that they wouldn't turn in. I straight out said I would not continue paying for tutoring if they received any more failing grades. I would send them to Lincoln's Challenge in Rantoul, Illinois, a program that helped with discipline and structure—two characteristics I felt they needed to learn. It was a difficult decision. I reached out to Mister again about helping them. We had agreed that once they reached the age of thirteen, they could live with him so he could give them what I couldn't provide as their mother. Regrettably, when the time came, Mister was incarcerated. I helped him get time off his sentence by writing a letter to the judge as he requested and sending the judge his certificate for a substance abuse class he took while incarcerated. Upon release, he said he barely had a place for himself, much less two boys. It hurt my heart once again for my sons, but I knew for certain that Mister was unreliable and unhelpful, and that would not change.

I prayed, I talked to God, I wrote in my journal. I spoke with Neon's neurologist and the psychologist to gather their opinions on sending the boys to Lincoln's Challenge. I received positive feedback. Because they continued failing, I kept my word and sent them to that school. Many criticized me negatively for my decision, but I held on to what God said. He knew I didn't want them to be away from me and our home. But I saw the path they were on, and I did not want that to continue. In December 2015, my twin Son shines graduated from Lincoln's Challenge. While neither could pass the GED exam, they were motivated to continue their learning and began taking adult learning classes at South Suburban College, then Prairie State. Deon went on to achieve his GED and attend Job Corps in Joliet, Illinois. He graduated with a concentration in Culinary Arts. Job Corps wouldn't accept Neon because they did not want responsibility for any epileptic seizures.

Against all odds, once again, the twins proved they can excel and achieve anything they put their minds to. I am so proud of my gentlemen—who they are and who they will become. Our journey was not simple and still has its challenges. But with work, obedience, sacrifice, love, and much prayer, good can prevail.

In the process, I became hardened, more masculine than I already was by default. I didn't choose to be a single mother, nor did I choose to be Superwoman. It was sink or swim—and I knew I could not sink with my children. Instead, I adapted, shifted, and redirected my energy to being the best mother I could be. It sounds so cliché and the pressure was indeed tremendous. Being a woman with a career in a male-dominated field like accounting was also extremely difficult. I had to earn their respect and show them I completely earned my position, my title, and my promotions. Colleagues questioned my bachelor's degree from an HBCU. Colleagues assumed I was an administrative assistant instead of an agent like them because of my race. I overlooked daily microaggressions from racist co-workers. In every location I worked, I managed to find my tribe of people who became allies and friends. I learned early, and out of necessity, to block out negativity and non-essential individuals as I steamed ahead to provide for and feed my children.

I worked every day under the weight of caretaking for three unique individuals other than myself *by myself*. I woke up each day determined to make their life better than mine. Since I knew sexual abuse, I had an awareness of the need to have conversations about sex early on with my Son-shines. I pushed education on them because I knew how it has helped change the trajectory of my life. I purposefully raised them in church knowing full well how my faith in God saved my life. All I have learned, I tried sharing with my sons—both the good and the bad. I didn't need to hide my shortcomings and mistakes from them so they could put me on a pedestal. I want them to see their parents as transparent, and certainly not perfect by any means. I never want them to aim for perfection because it is unattainable. We are all flawed and multidimensional.

Two conflicting facts can be true at the same time: I can be a good mother to my children but a bad wife to their father. For every good decision I made for their lives, I did it solo and rarely consulted their father. I never considered him as I graduated and moved from state to state in search of the best life for our children. I just naturally assumed since I was the breadwinner, it was my choice.

I never consulted him in choosing a pediatrician, a dentist, an education, a church. He was not part of building my house. We lead totally different lives. He refused to understand my evolution, and in truth, I didn't know him either. I had no clue about his life mission or his vision as a father. I had no knowledge of his fears, ambitions, and future goals—and vice versa. We met as college students from two parts of the world; at the time, we were both curious and lusting. We loved each other as much as a 19-year-old and a 20-year-old could.

We became pregnant by chance and had babies, now forced to make the best of it because we had become parents. As I faced my own expenses, I knew I could not depend on him nor even expect him to chip in because he had no consistent employment. In our thirteen years together, he never maintained a steady job for a year. It became a lonely existence for me not having a genuine partner—and in some ways, I'm sure he felt isolated as well. Sometimes I felt I had four children—Mister included.

I constantly imagined careers for him and supported his return to school while I worked. I was giving him grace to find himself without nagging about what I needed from him. I often wondered how our relationship would finally end, especially since he sometimes threatened my life if I ever left him and moved on. I prayed to God that I would be safe to raise my children, that no harm would befall me. When I found a chance to leave safely as a mutually agreed-upon decision to end our relationship, I took it and ran. Sadly, I didn't think me leaving him would result in him leaving our boys. It broke my heart seeing the boys waiting for someone who did not show up for a visit. He never came to see their sports games or choir concerts. I supplied Christmas and birthday presents for his sons by putting his name on the gifts. I thought we could at least maintain a friendship with some respect to co-parent our sons, but he showed me otherwise. Purposely tarnishing my name and sharing my childhood traumas with his harassing girlfriend were the last straws for me.

My main trial in being a single mother to three boys is how do I allow them to develop and grow on their own. I wanted them to stay close to me so I could help them, monitor them, and figure out their future for them. But after reading Steven Covey's book, *the 7 Habits of Highly Effective People*, I realized his wisdom: When we don't allow our children to develop on their own, we are communicating to them that they are not capable and need constant protection. If I didn't want to baby my sons forever, then I needed to change myself and my perception.

Therapy also provided great tools, such as journaling, to help me release my trauma. You cannot heal what you won't reveal. Just like Alice Walker's heroine in *The Color Purple*, Celie began each day with "Dear God," and that is how I start each day when I journal. I am an empath, so I carry everyone else's problems with mine. I actively try to help them in any way they need help. I paid for children's birthday parties that were not my own. I included people in my budget to make sure they didn't struggle even as I was struggling. This truly taught me who preferred my hand and not my heart. I had to learn how to release this pressure by praying for those individuals and giving the issue to God by writing it in my journal. It is all about how I placed my burdens down. I began using my journals as I would practice fasting throughout the years—forty-day periods most times. For forty days and nights, I would journal about issues, people, situations, and start ach page with "Dear God." Before the vision board craze, there was "Write the vision and make it plain." I described my vision, my mission, my goals, my hopes, my prayers, my dreams, my fears, and trusted God to handle them. Evidence of this was clear in my life: I went to college as if I had money and a financial plan, but I had no idea how to pay tuition. But I wanted my degree. Whatever I needed, I found the connection to earn the means to get what I needed, trusting God to do so. Nothing I did without faith, but I had to be willing to work with my mustard seed faith. I experienced great highs—my children's births, college graduation—and devastating lows—sexual abuse, divorce, single motherhood. I had achieved great successes—promotions and building a home—and awful losses—the deaths of so many precious family members and friends. But faith has remained steadfast through all of it.

I also have incredible fears, which are tangibly real African American males in our present-day climate of police brutality and injustice. Seeing Trayvon Martin, Oscar Grant, Laquan McDonald, Michael Brown, Alton Sterling, and countless other unarmed Black boys and men murdered by police officers affected me greatly. As Emmett Till's mom stated, when something happens to any of us, it is the business of all of us. I worry constantly for my young Black men. If I didn't know where they were and who they were with, my nervous system would scream. I had to learn how to close my eyes, inhale/exhale, breathe in the moment, smell the air around me, observe nature around me, and whisper "God is in control." I'm not sure if I can explain it, but when I feel I cannot control what happens on any given day, I run away in my mind to the next day for a better chance. Even when I read a book and I reach the climactic moment in the story, I must go to the last page to calm myself. I have had severe control issues because of my control over my body, and my choices were taken from me.

I barely remember my life before my boys. I must trust the way I raise them. I worked hard to embed values into their insides, their characters. They do not wear labels identifying them on their exteriors. I raised them in church so they would have their own personal relationship with God. I took them to annual physicals, whether the school required them or not. I took them to the dentist bi-annually and the orthodontist for braces. My conclusion is: There was no area of their well-being that I didn't consider as I raised them.

I considered their well-being through my faith that carried me through unprecedented storms. I found a church to fellowship within every city that was home. I attended Zion Traveler Baptist Church until I graduated from Grambling State University in July 2001. I attended Tried Stone Baptist Church in Cincinnati until moving back to Chicago in 2003. I attended Apostolic Church of God, where I was baptized as a child and my 7-year-old twins were baptized. In 2007, when we moved to Fort Wayne, we joined the Come as You Are Church. The fact remains: My faith guides me. I trust God. When I am lost, I go to God. My goal is no longer perfection but being true to who I am in whatever season I am in. I make no apologies and give no explanations for becoming whoever I needed to be to survive my storms. I have lied, cheated, gossiped, but I do not measure any of these since over any other. I strive to be my best self. I stay in my lane, driving towards my goals. Whoever shares my path will join me at the finish line for the victory lap.

MAKING FAITH MOVES

My great-grandmother took me to church with her as a child at the storefront on 67th & Ashland. My mother and Auntie Bettye took us to Apostolic Church of God on 6320 S. Dorchester. My cousin Charles took me to church with him as I grew up in Chicago. When I was in school in Louisiana, I attended Zion Traveler Baptist Church. No matter where I lived, I found my way to a church like iron filings flying to a magnet. My relationship with God was the only anchor that kept me sane most days. In Dr. Eric Thomas's book, *You Owe You*, he states, "But when I got to a church service, I felt embraced and seen and loved." I feel the same way. Dr. Thomas adds, "One of my strengths is that I'm a naturally positive person." I consider myself an authentically, intentionally positive person. That is, I make a conscious choice each waking day to be grateful and amazing, to be a light for others. What I discovered about myself is that I love being in the presence of elders to gain insights into life and wisdom. I love being in the presence of my peers for shared life experiences, laughter, and joy. And, of course, I love being in the presence of babies—my own and others—to breathe a fresh outlook on life and gain humility. I had resolved by this time that I was raising boys to become Men which meant, no matter what was thrown at me that I had to hold my head up, stick my chest out and handle it like Tupac stated in *Keep your head up*.

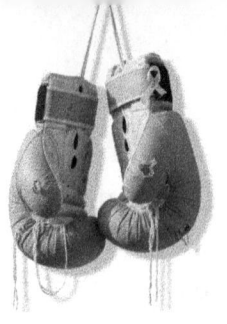

CHAPTER 7

Notorious B.I.G.:
"WE CAN'T CHANGE THE WORLD UNTIL WE CHANGE OURSELVES."

In 2001, when I was living in Cincinnati and going through so much, I used to drive somewhere by myself, park, and sit in my car, and cry alone. I listened to "You Are My Friend" by Patti LaBelle and reflect on the memories I shared with my cousin Karen. Her recent death left me feeling isolated in my grief and sorrow, and I profoundly missed our conversations. She was a safe place for me to share my feelings with.

I was so unhappy in my relationship and felt so alone. One of my favorite meditation techniques to clear my head was to take a nice ride down Lake Shore Drive in Chicago. I blasted songs as I drove, like "Paid in Full: by Eric B. and Rakim and songs by Mary Mary and Kirk Franklin. I am a lover of hip hop, preferably what they call classic or old school. Again, two opposing facts can be true simultaneously: I love hip hop, and I love the Lord. Some people might have a problem with that, but I don't let other people's issues become my issue. Just like Sanaa Lathan's character in *Brown Sugar*, hip hop music has been a first love that has changed my mood and set the tone when I need it.

In each season of my life, I have used reading books and scriptures and listening to music to help me navigate my storms. I began journal writing to help me heal and process. It was a therapeutic tool I learned from going to therapy. I introduced my twins to therapy when they began having behavior issues in school, which I knew was their way of expressing themselves in Mister's absence. I set up therapy for all of us to go, but the therapist told me I was wasting my time with Mister in therapy. It was obvious Mister wasn't interested in attending and didn't take it seriously. I paid for therapy for myself, for us, and for each child separately. I wanted them to use their voice and gain useful tools necessary for when they were going through a particularly rough time in life. I made sure we were all active members of our church. I made sure my boys had extra help with academics by taking them to Sylvan Learning Center for tutoring and educational assessment. I made sure my son had a pediatric neurologist and saw specialists as needed for his medical care. I put both in Karate classes to help with discipline.

They indulged in basketball, football, swimming, tennis, and golf in summer camp. Raising children is so much more than dressing them up. It is intentionally setting them up for their future, helping them become self-sufficient, and teaching them leadership, accountability, responsibility, and respectability. Parenting is giving love and support unconditionally, whether they choose the life you planned for them or not. So many times, I wanted to get revenge for how Mister treated our children with his absence. When Mister became incarcerated, I still took them to see him, write him letters, sent pictures of them, and even wrote to the judge on his behalf at his request. I just wanted us to coparent peacefully so the boys could experience the best parts of both of us.

Because I knew Mister's background and how he was raised, I always advised my children to give him grace, just as God gives us grace because we all make mistakes. I explained that their father's mother suffered from substance abuse, and I never met his father in the 13 years we were together. God kept my Son-shines and me together and strong through all the pain. I cried myself to sleep some nights from the exhaustion of all the responsibilities in my life. God was my only solace of hope. I placed my faith firmly in God's hands while raising my children. Or else I would have lost my mind.

I endured Mister weaponizing my childhood trauma against me to control me. I sustained a school principal weaponizing a state agency against me and my children to control us. Both were equally painful. I prayed to release the pain from my heart and strategize an escape from that toxicity.

My family ensured that I was raised in the church. When I raised my children, I took this a step further to include explaining *why* I was raising them in church. I had conversations with my children every Sunday after the service about the lesson they learned and how to use it in their lives. I tried to teach them that we attend church not for tradition or habit but for survival and sanity. When life gets difficult, I wanted them to go to God instead of alcohol, drugs, or any unhealthy growth. I realized the importance of seeking God during challenging times. I trusted that even if they fell, they fell on a solid foundation. I have fallen many times before. I used lures like sex, work, and shopping, but nothing helped. I learned through trial and error that God was where to go when trouble arose. I began a 40-day fasting journey, documenting each day in my journal and engaging in meditation and prayer. During this period, I also eliminated certain activities such as using social media, consuming junk food, or watching television. I continually challenged myself to be disciplined and stop any activity that was proving harmful, at least for a specified period.

I have learned grace and empathy for others through my life experiences. I know I have passed through many tests and trials, especially since raising my children. Unfortunately, they had to endure it all with me as I was working to discover who I was and what it meant to be their mother. This made me realize the same for my parents. I appreciate everything they did for me, including battling their own traumas while raising me as best they could. While raising my children, I accepted that they would inevitably also see and judge my struggles. I had twins at the age of 22 and, just like my parents, I was a young parent. I was especially hard on the twins because I had no reference on being a mother. I had Zion at the age of 30 and tried managing an unexpected event just as my parents did before me. No one escapes human experiences, regardless of one's degree of spirituality.

I apologize to my children for any harm I caused them while I raised them. We grew up together, and they taught me as much as I them. Everyone should put their parents in perspective. They are human too, may have had childhood traumas, and traveled both peaks and valleys. My children may have seen me struggle but they didn't see me give up, leave, or fold under pressure. I pray they follow the same example. Fall and stumble but always get back up.

I have never left my children, as I promised them the day, I met my twins at the NICU and my third child in my birth room. My mission as a parent has always been giving unconditional love, setting a solid foundation in God, teaching all I know, providing resources to become self-sufficient, allowing grace and space to grow, supporting them, encouraging their dreams, and being authentically transparent to them and myself.

I let them choose their dress, their styles. None of it matters if they are not great people. I never wanted them to be my carbon copy. Instead, I nurtured them to speak out and live their truth. I love to see the human beings God created them to be. I love them so much. I used to sit up for hours after putting them to sleep, thinking, planning, wondering what they would become, and worrying if I was a good parent. I sought ways to improve my listening to them, feeding them with opportunities. I dreamed of their success; however, they would need to define it. My legacy on earth began with them. I taught them about their world, their history, and God's place for them in this life. Every prayer I breathe with my heart and intentions has been, and will always be, for them.

Perspective can play a significant role in understanding generational differences. The upbringing of individuals from the baby boomer generation—those born between 1946 and 1964—was shaped by the experiences and values of their parents. Boomers are named for the population "boom" that occurred after WWII, and many young people of this generation defied their parents, protested the Vietnam War, and created the "Summer of Love." They raised their children with a focus on wanting the best for them and both parents worked. Making sure their children went to college was a priority that wasn't in the generation before them. Their demographic could not be more different from The Silent Generation who raised them and that shows in their parenting styles. This generation cared about the perspective of how kids felt growing up. Gen Xers are all about parenting. They are a generation that focuses on learning about parenting and caring about work-life balance. They understand the importance of individualism and tend to support their children's choices for different lifestyles more than past generations. Generation X is also a generation of volunteers and are very involved in their kids' development. Generation X covers those born between 1965 to 1980. We were the first latchkey kids, very independent from a very young age. Generation X demonstrates a strong commitment to parenting, with an emphasis on educating themselves regarding effective parenting strategies and maintaining a healthy work-life balance. This generation values individualism and is generally more supportive of their children's diverse lifestyle choices compared to previous generations. Generation X is also a generation of volunteers and are very involved in their kids' development. As a parent, I used the knowledge I learned from how my parents raised me to raise my own children.

Making Faith Moves: I stayed with Mister to try to save the little boy inside of him that had similar trauma to mine in hopes that maybe one day he would save the little girl inside of me. Once I realized he would not or could not, it was painful, but I knew it was over. Change began with me. Like Michael Jackson sang, I had to look at the woman in the mirror. I had to be humble enough to apologize for the way I behaved when I was acting from a place of trauma and change without excuses. I recognized the importance of acknowledging my shortcomings and learning from them, emphasizing both accountability and responsibility. Meaningful change—whether within myself or in my surroundings—required introspection, self-awareness, and a commitment to personal growth and healing.

PTSD after sexual assault is a deeply painful and complex experience, and you're not alone in facing it. Survivors often experience a range of symptoms that can affect their emotional, mental, and even physical health—sometimes for months or years if left untreated.

Common PTSD Symptoms After Sexual Assault

Flashbacks and nightmares: Reliving the trauma through vivid memories or dreams

Hypervigilance: Feeling constantly on edge or unsafe, even in familiar environments

Avoidance: Steering clear of places, people, or conversations that remind you of the event

Emotional numbness or dissociation: Feeling disconnected from yourself or your surroundings

Guilt, shame, or self-blame: Even though the survivor is never at fault, these feelings are tragically common

Having difficulty trusting others: Especially in relationships or social situations

Treatment and Support Options

Trauma-focused therapy: Approaches like EMDR (Eye Movement Desensitization and Reprocessing) or CBT (Cognitive Behavioral Therapy) have shown strong results

Medication: Antidepressants or anti-anxiety medications may help manage symptoms, but should be discussed with a psychiatrist

Support groups: Connecting with others who've had similar experiences can be incredibly validating and healing

Online therapy platforms: These can offer accessible care, especially if in-person options feel overwhelming

Crisis and Support Resources

If you or someone you know is in immediate need:

RAINN (U.S.): 1-800-656-HOPE or rainn.org

Crisis Text Line: Text HOME to 741741

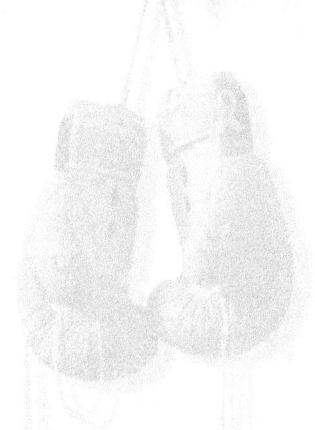

PART II

THE DEGREE — THE MISEDUCATION OF SANDY, USING MY FAITH TO ESCAPE POVERTY

> Chinese philosopher Lao Tzu once said:
>
> *Give a man a fish and you feed him for a day. Teach him how to fish and you feed him for a lifetime.*

I can do all things through Christ which strengthened me.
Phil. 4:13

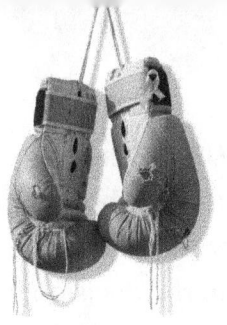

CHAPTER 8

Malcolm X:
"EDUCATION IS OUR PASSPORT TO THE FUTURE, FOR TOMORROW BELONGS TO THE PEOPLE WHO PREPARE FOR IT TODAY."

In 1954, a year before my mother was born, the groundbreaking case, Brown v. Board of Education of Topeka sparked the nation. This was a landmark decision of the United States Supreme Court which ruled that U.S. state laws establishing racial segregation in public schools violate the Equal Protection Clause of the Fourteenth Amendment and hence are unconstitutional, even if the segregated facilities are presumed to be equal.

The Court's unanimous decision in Brown and its related cases paved the way for integration and was a major victory of the civil rights movement. A special three-judge court of the U.S. District Court for the District of Kansas heard the case and ruled against the Browns, relying on the precedent of Plessy and its "separate but equal" doctrine. The Browns, represented by NAACP chief counsel Thurgood Marshall, appealed the ruling directly to the Supreme Court, who issued a unanimous 9–0 decision in favor of the Browns. On May 17, 1954, the Supreme Court laid out a new precedent: Separate but equal has no place in American schools. The message from Brown v. Board of Education was clear. But 70 years later, the impact of the decision is still up for debate.

When I was around ten years old, I read the *Autobiography of Malcolm X* as told to Alex Haley. It changed my life. Malcolm X's book inspired me and opened my eyes to consciousness. I learned the history of Blacks in America from a different lens. This book introduced me to Marcus Garvey through Malcolm X's father, Earl Little, following Garvey's teachings. I instantly became intrigued to learn more about African American leaders since school so far had only introduced me to Dr. Martin Luther King, Jr., because he was "safe" to the powers-that-be that approved the elementary education curriculum—that is, he preached non-violence, ironically, he was later assassinated, his brother was murdered and his mother. This infuriated me to think how much other people hate African American people and portray us as violent. I researched books about Frederick Douglass, Harriet Tubman, Sojourner Truth, Ida B. Wells, and Nat Turner. I also read books by brilliant authors such as Nikki Giovanni, James Baldwin, Toni Morrison, and Maya Angelou.

- "Knowledge makes a man unfit to be a slave." Frederick Douglass

The more I read and comprehended how my royal ancestors were kidnapped from their own land, brought to America in deplorable conditions, enslaved, forced to work for nothing, abused, raped, kidnapped, beaten, and murdered for any reason, including rights they should have had such as learning, the more I was enlightened on our struggles in America. While I was horrified, I admired their strength to better themselves and future generations under the worst conditions. They remained here after slavery was abolished in the United States and built the cotton industry, railroads, infrastructures, and even the White House just to name a few. Black women were made to cook, clean homes, raise the children of their owners while being treated like animals and raped to bear children for their Massa. None of these children were claimed or recognized by these white men.

A woman named Isabella changed her name to Sojourner Truth and spoke truth to power. I am inspired by women like Nina Simone and Billie Holiday who would not keep quiet about the travesties happening to Black people. Reading about these heroes and heroines made me want to succeed not just for myself and my family, but also for my community and culture. I wanted to honor their legacies by joining their plight in my way, using my God-given gifts according to my purpose. I was now evolving into a mentality of including others besides myself. No longer thinking of what my community can do for me, now I began thinking about how I could help my community. That's when I realized I loved reading and writing poetry.

I hate tormentors and always protected those I felt couldn't or wouldn't use their voices, not for fear of physical harm necessarily but for fear of mental or emotional harm. I use my knowledge to speak up and speak out against any form of bullying. This is why as a child I wanted to become a lawyer. The Phylicia Rashad character, Claire Huxtable, on *The Cosby Show*, reminded me of my mother—smart, sharp dresser, no-nonsense, beautiful wife, mother and attorney. She was respected and took no mess, like my mother. I began saying to anyone who asked that I wanted to grow up to be an attorney, like Claire Huxtable.

I realized then how important knowledge was, and once achieved, it cannot be taken away from you. By the time I was a teenager, I learned of poet and rapper Tupac Shakur, who spoke out about injustices happening to my culture. He had a bold voice and talent.

His parents were Black Panthers, active in the movement of equality for Black people. Tupac was the type of artist who used his influence to oppose harassment of any kind. When I saw him on one of my favorite shows, A *Different World*, I adored him even more for the selection of projects he chose to join. A *Different World* influenced my decision to attend a Historically Black College and University (HBCU). Originating back to the 19th century, HBCUs were created by our ancestors who could not get acceptance into the established colleges or universities, so they began their own to offer Black students opportunities for higher education.

I loved learning, reading books, writing stories, and socializing. School fascinated me. I identify as an introverted extrovert, also called an "outgoing introvert" or "ambivert," someone who enjoys social interaction but needs time alone to recharge. I wanted attention but not too much where I couldn't blend in. However, my grades were above average, and teachers pursued me to apply to math competitions, spelling bees, or junior author contests. I would get far enough to win in my class or grade but then stopped short. I purposely lost the school battle. I did not want to represent my school for fear of standing out. I still recall the word I misspelled in the spelling bee: "Scorpion." I spelled it s-c-o-r-p-i-A-n on purpose. I wrote short stories, essays, and poetry and entered the junior author contest. I can still remember the story that I wrote that my teacher, Mrs. Wright, submitted. It was good, but not enough to be featured in our local newspaper. I planned it that way because I did not want to win.

When I was in elementary school, I developed my love for reading. I read the books my mother had at home like *The Color Purple* by Alice Walker. I read Joan Collins, John Grisham, James Patterson, and V. C. Andrews. All these books, along with The Coldest Winter

Ever by Sista Soulja that I read as a teenager, opened my mind and taught me more about the world. Their narration and characters I felt were so remarkable. I learned so much from Nikki Giovanni, Toni Morrison, and Maya Angelou about the trials and triumphs of being a Black woman. These well-educated women had traveled the world and had so much to say, so I wanted to see the world as they described it. I too wanted to travel the world and write stories; create characters people could identify with and root for. Reading became my escape like music. I loved a good story, whether it took the form of a book or a dope beat. I marveled at artists who expressed themselves with their creativity.

My seventh grade Iowa test scores were high enough that I could choose the high school I wanted and not be confined to my neighborhood high school. I chose Hyde Park Career Academy since my brother and cousin attended it at the time, and my parents graduated from it as well. It was in my old neighborhood, Woodlawn, so I already knew some people there. The summer of 1990, I graduated eighth grade, and my mother bought her first house—a two-story, three-bedroom/1.5 bath townhouse over east near 79th Colfax. We were so happy to be moving on up in the world. My father lived nearby with his girlfriend and her baby girl at this time.

By now I was a pro at catching the bus, and it took two buses one way to arrive at Hyde Park Career Academy from my mom's house. Even though my brother and I were now attending the same school, we didn't travel together. He usually left earlier and stayed after school for track or football. My mother gave me "car fare"—usually tokens—because the bus fare is half off for students and my mother would buy like a month's worth of tokens. I walked to the bus stop in the morning from 81st Colfax to 79th Colfax, cross the street for the 79th Street bus going west, pay my fare and find a seat (or stand) until either Stony Island or Jeffrey. Then, I waited for another bus to take me to 62nd Stony Island, where Hyde Park was located.

Since Hyde Park was not my local high school, I enrolled in their college preparatory magnet program which meant that all my classes were honors except lunch and gym, and I had no classes with regular high school students. To go to Hyde Park, I had to be in the college prep program or magnet program for academically above average students.

After school was over for the day, most students at Hyde Park Career Academy walked to the bus stop on Stony Island in the direction of our homes. Violence surrounded us, and we had to be careful of hanging out with the wrong people and always being aware. One time, a guy was shot on the 63rd Street bus, and another time, a guy got beat up by a rival gang and pushed off the moving bus. We saw both females and males get jumped on by gang members—the term for which was "mob action."

My lunch crew at Hyde Park—Kim, Jafrika, Pam, Tekeia, Belinda, Billie Jean, and Lisa—had so much fun hanging outside in the park across from the school in the spring. It was at Hyde Park that I met so many friends that I still cherish this day.

My boyfriend, Jay, was back in the county jail for the second time, so he couldn't pick me up from school. One day, in my junior year, I was walking to the bus stop with a friend of mine, Naishon. As we waited, a guy in a nice car across the street called my name. I noticed it was Lucifer (a pseudonym), whom I had met a few days before walking down 71st Street who happened to be my cousin's boyfriend, which meant off limits for dating me. Plus, he wasn't my type! I waved back at him and continued standing with Naishon waiting for my girl Ketari to come by. Lucifer made a U-turn and pulled up in front of us. Another guy in the car with him.

Lucifer: *Where were you headed?*

Me: *Home on 80th Colfax.*

Lucifer: *I'll give you a ride, I'm going that way.*

Me: *No, I'm cool, I don't want to leave my girl.*

Lucifer: *Where is she going?*

Naishon: *On 80th Crandon.*

Lucifer: *That's cool. I can drop both of y'all off.*

I had a funny feeling, but I blew it off because Naishon was with me. We stopped at the Checkers Restaurant to eat, then dropped Naishon off first because her house was on the way to mine. Lucifer's pager went off, so he asked if I minded if he went to his grandmother's house to use her phone right away quickly. I shrugged while munching on Checkers fries. He pulled up at this house across the street from South Shore High School. He and his friend got out, and he told me to switch to the front seat. I listened to hip hop from the booming speakers when he came back and asked me to come with him into his grandmother's house because he was waiting for a call. It was nicely finished—sort of old-person nice where the furniture was white and covered in plastic. He directed me to the bedroom and turned on music videos, then left. I began to feel nervous, scanning the room to see if I could find something to use as a weapon, just in case. After ten minutes, he came in, pulling me up with my hands and mentioning how pretty I looked. I reminded him he was with my cousin, and we don't do that. I asked him to take me home and I reached for the doorknob.

Suddenly, he snapped. He said he wasn't playing with my little skinny ass, and I should lie down. He raised his hand as if to strike me. He looked so evil at that moment. I froze, and he shoved me onto the huge bed. He pulled down my pants, cussing me, and then violently entered me. It felt like hours of torture, but it was only four minutes. I watched the clock: 4:13 to 4:17. Strange what one remembers in trauma. When he finished, he told me to pull my pants up so we could go. He blasted "Pocketful of Stones" by UGK as he drove me home. Even though I was a fan of UGK, I could not listen to that song for more than ten years after I was in therapy. I don't remember the ride to my house. I don't remember who was home when I opened the door. I went to the bathroom and showered my numb body. I was too shocked to cry, so once again, I internalized my pain. I was disgusted. I scrubbed my body, as if I could erase the rape, erase his smell on my skin.

I went through the gamut of emotions such as fear, shame, humiliation, guilt, and self-blame which are common for sexual abuse victims and can lead to depression and anxiety. I experienced intrusive or recurring thoughts of abuse as well as nightmares or flashbacks. Most survivors of sexual abuse, including myself, often develop a belief that they caused the sexual abuse and that they deserved it.

Lucifer had the audacity to call me that night. His voice alone frightened me. It was a short conversation. He said if I told anyone what happened, he would tell my cousin I came up to him. I didn't want my cousin to have to choose between him and me. I had no intention of telling anyone but the Lord. I knew if I told my family, Lucifer would be handled by street justice, and I didn't want Jay or my family to end up in jail or worse. I felt responsible for protecting my family from this. I later learned Lucifer had a reputation for physical abuse and rape. He did the same to someone else I knew. Lucifer was murdered in 2001.

This became one of my worst semesters. I was just doing the bare minimum simply to cope. My grades fell to Cs and Ds. I was so ashamed I even tried changing my report card, wetting it so I could trace over the bad letters. But my mother detected it right away. I promised to do better, but I didn't care anymore. My mind was running all over, and I could not understand my teenage emotions.

I had secretly worried that I had contracted some lifelong disease from being raped at 16 years of age. Unfortunately, after the rape, I became more sexually active and found I could detach my emotions from the act of sex. I had a low regard of males. I assumed all males were the same, and if I found myself alone with one, they will take what they want anyway, so I might as well just give it over. Part of me surrounded myself with people so I wouldn't be alone with men. Sex and relationships became my vice—from the age of 13 until about 32. I kept what I used to call a "bench-full" of guys waiting to date me on standby, in case my official boyfriend wasn't keeping me happy or doing stuff I didn't like. I kept in touch with my "bench" just enough to sustain their interest in me. It was my way of protecting my heart from involvement with anyone who would, no doubt, break my heart. I dated like a chain smoker, ending one relationship while lighting up the next. Dating was never my focus, just something I did with whoever I chose for as long as I chose. Everyone was disposable. Until I became a mother. It was then that two little vulnerable men taught me unconditional love, patience, grace, and mercy, not just in words but in action.

I was already not craving attention for being too smart, cute, or popular. Now I wanted to shrink and fade into oblivion. Men were untrustworthy, and I felt I had to hurt them before they hurt me.

I began a vicious cycle of becoming nonchalant about my feelings towards males, especially in relationships. I was numb. I wanted to leave Chicago for a college far away because I no longer felt safe or protected and wanted to experience something different. I needed to change my environment.

I sat in my room by myself reading books and writing poetry. I didn't want to go outside and hang out anymore. After the rape, I became cold and aloof, especially about dudes. If I went out, it would be in groups because I didn't trust a guy alone. In my time, guys were always hollering, "Bro's before hoes," especially in Chicago where most guys thought they were pimps and treated females as disposable. So, I treated them the same way. I believed that for a female to be "pimpish," she had to finesse a guy into buying her stuff without giving up her body.

I began saying I would never get married or have children because I didn't want that level of commitment to a man. My hurt began a cycle of self-destruction. My mind raced with thoughts of horrible incidents that could happen because I was raped. I watched movies all the time, especially on Lifetime Network, where women caught a disease or became barren from being raped. Would I get an STD or HIV/AIDS? Will I be able to have children? These thoughts terrified me.

In Spring 1993, my junior year of high school, I went with a male friend to his senior prom and didn't tell my boyfriend, Jay, about it. I knew he wouldn't like it. Jay was locked up in the county jail when I went to the prom. After he got out of jail and started picking me up again, I hid that prom picture from him on display in my mother's living room.

Eventually, Jay's lifestyle turned me off. I didn't want to date a drug dealer, gang banger, or anyone growing up in the hood on the

Southside of Chicago. I had seen my fair share of female friends and classmates get caught up in a bad life because of their man—dealing with other women chasing after him because of his money and power, caught in shootouts, armed robberies, all sorts of abuse. I knew that life was not for me. I couldn't win living that life. Although I knew people in gangs, I but never got initiated into one. I knew enough about them to stay safe. I didn't want everyone's attention because a drug dealer or gangbanger was buying me all the flyest gear. Back then we wore Used jeans, Cross Color, Karl Kani, Girbaud, Guess, Fila, Coach, and carried an Eddie Bauer portfolio or bookbag to be cool. We listened to rappers like Twista, Psychodrama, Tupac, The Dogg Pound, and Crucial Conflict. Most of our communities didn't have field houses or recreational centers for young people to hang, so we stayed in our neighborhoods. We sat on porches watching people drive or walk by. We cracked jokes, danced, made up songs, rapped, or talked about our future.

Growing up in the city, you earned a reputation for being able to fight. You earned your stripes for kicking butt, male or female. You earned a rep for being a fly guy or girl with the latest and best gear. You had to have on name-brand clothes, shoes, and purses—exclusive stuff only so you can be like, "you don't know about this..." Those possessions got you notoriety for growing up where I'm from. Not for being smart back then. It is possible to be smart and cool. I refused to do what was expected of me, according to the negative stereotypes of black people in the world.

Historically, Black women used hairstyles to escape by weaving maps and coded messages into their braids, which allowed them to communicate and navigate their routes to freedom. These intricate styles could represent escape routes, signal a desire to flee, or even hide essential resources like seeds and gold. Since enslaved people were often forbidden to read or write, hair was a method of communication to pass information and keep it from enslavers. In 1786, the Spanish governor of Louisiana enacted the "tignon law," requiring women of African descent, both enslaved and free, to cover their hair with a knotted headdress. The law was intended to shame Black women and devalue their social status, partly because their ornate hair adornments were seen as a threat to white women.

Every Friday night and all-day Saturdays, barbershops and beauty shops were filled with black people trying to look their best. Black women stayed in beauty shop for hours getting our hair styled. We would maintain our hair style by sleeping delicately. We refused to exercise or do anything to mess up our hair style to the point of me jeopardizing my grade point average by not participating in swim class in high school. My beautician and hair stylist's name was Paulette and her assistant's name was Trivia. They were an awesome team since I was 16 years old, I followed wherever she did hair because she did my hair the best. I went to the beauty shop twice a month or every other week. Back in the 90's only people that wore wigs were our grandmothers, we didn't exaggerate baby hair, we were heavy on being natural, wearing our own hair without weaves and extensions. Men would tease women if they wore weaves by calling it horsehair, so we took pride in our hair.

The Crown Act was created in 2019 by Dove and the CROWN Coalition, in partnership with then State Senator Holly J. Mitchell of California, to ensure protection against discrimination based on race-based hairstyles by extending statutory protection to hair texture and protective styles such as braids, locs, twists, and knots in the workplace and public schools.

Our communities in the city were filled with liquor stores, unhealthy food choices, high-interest lending institutions, predatory businesses, abandoned buildings, and homes boarded up intentionally. Most of these wrecks were a result of redlining and white flight. Like Tupac said, we are not meant to survive because, it's a setup, speaking on systematic racism in every facet of black lives. When Black Americans began moving into neighborhoods with white Americans, the whites began moving out—particularly from those urban areas with significant minority populations—and escaped to the suburbs.

The Housing Act of 1937, also known as the Wagner–Steagall Act, provided federal subsidies to local public housing agencies (LHAs) in the United States. These subsidies aimed to improve living conditions for low-income families by supporting the construction and maintenance of public housing. Public housing—or what we call the projects, like Cabrini-Green and Ida B. Wells—was for low-income families. We used to have good times visiting relatives in those buildings, but the intention of the developers was for residents to live like prisoners in these run-down buildings. The intention of this "project" was to house black Americans in these housing situations surrounded by liquor stores and low wages. Drugs and guns were purposely dropped into these communities for us to get drunk, use drugs and kill each other.

Chicago is mostly segregated, we have the southside ad westside that are mostly populated by black people, we have little Italy, Chinatown, etc., Redlining is an illegal discriminatory practice that puts financial services—out of reach for residents of certain areas based on race or ethnicity. The term "redlining" was coined by sociologist John McKnight in the 1960s and is derived from the practice—used by the federal government and lenders—of literally drawing a red line on a map around the neighborhoods in which they would not invest, based on demographics alone. Black, inner-city neighborhoods were most likely to be redlined. Investigations found that lenders made loans to lower-income white borrowers but not to middle- or upper-income Black borrowers. In 1968, The Fair Housing Act was passed; it was federal legislation that protected individuals and families from discrimination in the sale, rental, financing, or advertising of housing. This Act forbade discrimination against minorities by real estate brokers, property owners, and landlords. The Home Mortgage Disclosure Act (HMDA) of 1975 required lending institutions to report public loan data, while the Community Reinvestment Act of 1977 was intended to encourage banks and other financial institutions to meet the credit needs of the communities in which they operate. The Fair Housing Act, amended in 1988, prohibits discrimination based on race, color, religion, sex, disability, family status, and national origin.

The police constantly came by to harass us in our communities, routinely checking for drugs and even planting drugs on one of my friends from the neighborhood. However, since we were all outside and saw the officer pull the drugs from his jacket, he played it off as a joke. The police often beat up guys who were just standing around if they asked a question or showed an attitude. There would be no help in this case. Who do you call for help against the police? This partially explains our relationship with the police in our communities: We don't trust them, and they don't respect us.

This history stemmed from the origin of police officers working as a slave patrol, authorities who essentially stopped every Black person to check their freedom papers and let them know they were beneath them. Wikipedia defines slave patrols (also known as paddy rollers)

as organized groups of armed men who monitored and enforced discipline upon slaves in the antebellum U.S. southern states. The slave patrols' function was to police slaves, especially those who escaped or were viewed as defiant. They also formed river patrols to prevent escape by boat. Slave patrols were first established in South Carolina in 1704, and the idea spread throughout the colonies before their use ended following the Civil War.

The South lost the Civil War, but white Americans stressed they feared Black Americans enough to practice lynching. They still practice lynching now, but they call it suicide. In the aftermath of the war, informal patrols sprang into action. Later, city and rural police squads, along with the help of Union army officers, revived patrolling practices among free men. During the Reconstruction period of 1865 to 1877, old-style patrol methods resurfaced and were enforced by postwar Southern police officers and organizations such as the Ku Klux Klan.

This practice continues today with assertions like the stop-and-frisk practice used in most large cities. The police can stop somebody they think may have committed a crime or will commit a crime. They are also entitled to pat the individual down to determine if they have any weapons on their person. This is done at a higher rate to Black Americans. White Americans are aware of this practice and use it to their privilege, as in the case of white people calling the police on Black Americans for something as simple as bird watching or jogging in their area. They know that any interaction police officers have with Black Americans can become a tragedy. Just as I avoided drug dealers, pimps, and gangs in Chicago, I also bypassed interactions with the Chicago police.

Growing up, I didn't want to depend on anyone for what I wanted for my life. I knew then that I needed to establish a high-paying career and, so, that meant going to college. My mother tried to teach me how to cook, but I never wanted to learn, and Grandma Janet would get so upset with my resistance. I would retort, "I'm *gonna make money, Grandma. Somebody is gonna be cooking for me! I'm going to college so I can make my own money.*

For this reason and more, I KNEW I needed to focus on college and be around people with the same mindset. In the summer before my senior year, I began dating Anthony after I ended my four-year relationship with Jay for good. Anthony was smart and funny and heading somewhere in life. We went to senior prom together and spent most days with each other in our last year of high school. I loved his mother, sister, and family because they reminded me of my own family.

My mother and stepfather, Larry, struggled to pay all my senior fees. My father was getting remarried in 1994, so he didn't help financially. We pulled it together as usual, and I attended all my senior events looking good. My sister Jeanette usually attended all my senior events with me except prom, people even thought she was graduating with us. We would travel to high school together daily, sometimes we called a livery cab instead of taking the bus when it was too cold outside for us to be standing at a bus stop. My cousin Tee and I would meet up after school to exchange clothes, I would bring her my Girbaud outfits in exchange for her Guess outfits. Since we were the skinny girls in the family and lived in separate parts of the city and attended different high schools no one knew we shared trendy outfits.

Anthony applied and got accepted into many colleges, but I only applied to Grambling State University which my big brother attended. My brother's father, Moochie, took me to visit Grambling State in the spring of my senior year and I fell in love immediately when I saw Black people like me going to school, furthering their education, investing in establishing a career or a better life. The love and empowerment I felt once I stepped onto that campus were amazing.

I felt safe. I knew that was where I wanted to be, no matter what I needed to do to get there. When it came time to graduate high school, I applied. Grambling State University accepted me as a student in the fall of 1994.

That summer, I hung out mostly with Anthony, my sister Jeanette, my cousin Tinesha, and my cousin Tee. Most of the dates Anthony took me on were the movies which Jeanette and Tinesha usually came with us. Karen would spend the night at my mom's house and together all of us would make up dances and have talent shows to keep us entertained. Karen was five years younger than me, so she was like all our baby sisters, not just Terry, Jobe and Alex sister. I protected her fiercely and loved bossing her around, so much that she nicknamed me Angelica from the Rugrats. She told me I was her role model and I took that seriously, I never wanted to disappoint her.

I tried thinking about what I needed for college and purchased some necessities. I was nervous, excited, and anxious about this transition. I certainly didn't know what to expect. I was stepping out of my comfort zone. I left my parents, siblings, cousins, aunts, uncles, family, and friends to pursue something I only saw in my mind. I left my church, Apostolic Church of God, which I attended since I was a little girl along with my mother, my siblings, Auntie Bettye, and my first cousins, Terry, Tinesha, Tee, Stevie, Marcus, and Hollis.

I wanted to make my family proud. I dreamed of getting a degree, making good money, buying a house, and traveling the world. I wanted to come back and live in a Chicago neighborhood surrounded by my people, so other girls and boys sharing my background could see and know it is possible to go away to college and graduate.

As Sam Cooke sang, "A change is gonna come." That is how I felt. A change was coming. Leaving my beautiful city to attend college was exciting and overwhelming, but I was on a mission. I had a love/hate relationship with Chicago at that point. I had learned to observe and adjust to the changing seasons and being flexible through all weather conditions. One of the main reasons I loved Chicago is we had four seasons. Chicagoans endure brutal winters and cold fall seasons to get to the blossoms of spring and fun summertime Chi. Looking at the changing seasons always gave me hope. Seeing the bare trees in the winter covered with frost and ice and then watching them return in the spring taught me (as my Uncle Jobe used to say): "Tough times don't last, tough people do."

MAKING FAITH MOVES

Richard Wurmbrand said, "Faith is never passive. It demands a response. It asks for a mission." My mission was clear: find a way to take care of yourself and live the lifestyle you want. Like Kanye West said, everything I'm not makes me everything I am. I am not a boxer, a gangbanger, the flyest dressed, an athlete, or most popular. I am a nerd, so my way of completing my mission was through education. I had to navigate a plan through higher learning to establish my career and live the life I desired. I know I am a natural-born leader by the drive that exists within.

Dr. Martin Luther King, Jr., once said, "We need leaders not in love with money but in love with justice. Not in love with publicity but in love with humanity." My vision was not based on simply getting rich for the sake of having money, I am not greedy. My vision did not include wanting fame or popularity just to make people like me. I desired to gain wealth for myself, my family, my friends, and my community. I am a philanthropist, always giving back to my culture in whatever way I can. I never wanted to fit in because I know I stand out as leaders do and use my voice against injustice.

Decide for yourself what talents come naturally to you and follow that path. Prepare yourself for your path to success and wait for the opportunities to come. I had to figure out my educational path, prepare my mind for the journey no matter what the circumstance.

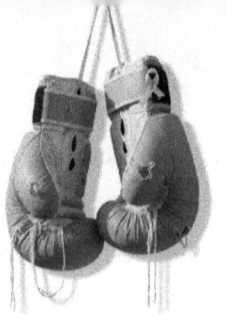

CHAPTER 9

Gwendolyn Brooks:
"DO NOT DESIRE TO FIT IN. DESIRE TO OBLIGE YOURSELVES TO LEAD."

It is possible to make it out of the hood without selling my soul, and I was going to prove it. I figured out the lifestyle I desired to live and knew it would take some money. I knew all the traps set up for people who looked like me coming from inner-city living. They want you to do something criminal to lock you up in the criminal justice system and become their slave, as per the 13th Amendment.

The 13th Amendment to the U.S. Constitution, ratified in 1865 in the aftermath of the Civil War, abolished slavery in the United States. The 13th Amendment states: "Neither slavery nor involuntary servitude, except as a punishment for crime whereof the party shall have been duly convicted, shall exist within the United States, or any place subject to their jurisdiction." This meant they ended slavery—except for criminals. I think of one of my favorite movies, *Life*, with brilliant comedians Eddie Murphy and Martin Lawrence. This movie depicts a story of two Black men from New York City who travel down South for a business proposition. Along the way, they get framed for murder by a white local sheriff and sentenced to life in Mississippi. They spend most of their life behind bars building railroads and other infrastructures for free as convicted criminals. Once you are trapped in the criminal justice system, it is hard to get out, even when you are innocent. I cautiously avoided criminal activity.

I was on my way to college in August 1994. My mother bought me a big TV for my dorm room and a comforter set. My father gave me some money. My brother Lonzo was already in Louisiana, so I rode with Anthony, his mother, and his sister to Grambling in August to begin my college life. I am still forever grateful to his mother, Ms. Idella, and sister, Tanara, for transporting me to school and being there for me as I embarked on my new journey. We rode in a packed van with all our belongings to move in our dorms. Even the air smelled different when we arrived at Grambling on Louisiana highway exit 81. I didn't know much about college, besides what I saw in the movie *School Daze* by Spike Lee and the TV show *A Different World*. My first thought was I would become roommates with my brother, instead of living in dorms with strangers. However, the rule was that freshmen had to stay in a dorm their first year. So, I applied for my dorm assignment late and had to take whatever they could find. I was assigned to Jones Hall, 4th floor.

I had to learn about registration, admissions, housing, classes, financial aid, and eating in the cafeteria. I had to figure out my day-to-day routine in a whole new place on a meager budget. My brother showed us around to register and complete the financial aid process. I found out how much we owed once all the aid was applied. Ms. Idella also helped us complete our registration and enrollment. I signed up for work-study because I didn't have enough loans and grants to cover my first year, even with the help of my parents. I chose to work in the admissions office. Work-study meant I worked a job but instead of earning a salary, the wages went to the school to cover tuition, room, and board. I signed up for work-study in addition to student loans and a Pell grant, and my balance due was a little over $100—may seem small today, but at that time, it was difficult to get even that much from my parents. Despite working hard, they just didn't earn enough—as was the case for most Black Americans. That's when I realized I was poor. My mother even took out a parent-plus loan to help.

When I moved into my dorm room with my clothes, TV, and comforter bedding, I found a huge cockroach at the door. And it flew! I had never seen flying roaches until moving to Louisiana. My dorm roommate was named Amita, a tall young woman from Bunkie, Louisiana. Her side of the room looked nice and coordinated. She introduced me to her cousin, Shonka, and their friends, Tylynn and Shay. Tylynn stayed down the hall from us on the 4th floor, with her roommate, Alison, from Newelton, Louisiana. Shay's room was on the 2nd floor. My next-door neighbor was a girl from the DMV (DC, Maryland, Virginia) area named Kelli, who was on the track team with my brother. First, they were friends, then she became my friend.

During my first night sleeping in my Louisiana dorm room, I remember closing my eyes as I lay on my twin-size dorm bed. I heard a peculiar noise. It was disturbing. I asked my roommate about it. *"What noise?"* she asked. *"Crickets?"* I guess so, I answered, moving over to the dorm window. Yes, that was the noise I was hearing. Amita was amazed I had never heard crickets. I told her I was from Chicago—no crickets at night on my block. There were the sounds of city life: You hear city life, loud music, cars, arguments, fighting, gunshots, ambulances, fire trucks, and police sirens at night. I loved it and had no crickets. My goodness—and seeing the stars in the

Louisiana night sky was magical. I constantly got lost looking at the stars at night. Chicago has too many streetlights to see the sky.

I began my classes as a Business Management major. I knew I didn't want to work in the healthcare field, and as much as I loved writing, I wasn't sure how it could be a career making good money right out of college. I figured I would need an advanced degree plus make the necessary contacts to establish myself as a journalist or writer. I wasn't interested in engineering or mass communications either. I made my choice based on careers I was *not* interested in and thus figured out what I wanted to do.

Most of my first-semester courses were mandatory freshman-level classes. I had two courses at Business College: Business Management and Accounting 101. I remember my boyfriend Anthony looking at my schedule and suggested I should not take Accounting because it was too hard for him. I thought to myself, "You're just not smart enough to handle that class!" You know what I did? I decided to make accounting my major. I was intrigued by the challenge it presented, and I don't back down from a challenge, especially about my intelligence. In my Accounting class, I saw a girl dressed as we did in Chicago back in the 1990s: oversized shorts, a cute hairstyle, and earrings with the Nike check but instead of Nike, they had her name, I'Esha. I asked her where she was from, and she confirmed it: Chicago! I told her my name and my hometown. We exchanged dorm room information before parting ways after class.

My first year, I mostly hung out with Anthony, my brother, and his friends. Most of the guys were from Texas who were used to partying a lot. I tagged along. Sometimes my dorm roommate and her friends come out and hang out with us too. Lots of drinking went on, but I didn't like beer or alcohol, I just listened to music, cracked jokes, and ate. The reality was that I was now living life on my own. No one here was setting a curfew. I had to learn how to balance my partying with my education. I had freedom except for having my boyfriend there. We were together every day after classes, and I started to feel almost married. Ironic that I had just left behind answering my parents, and now I was answering him. I had a feeling this wasn't going to work for very long.

My classes were interesting but challenging. I had to transition from being a high school student who did the bare minimum to thriving as a college student. I didn't know that attendance was a part of the grade for the first two years, so you *must* go to class to pass with a good grade. By my senior year of high school, I had begun a bad habit of cutting classes and only going to hand in assignments and take tests. So, when I received my first-semester college grades, I quickly understood how much attendance affected my grades. I incorrectly assumed if I just completed assignments and passed tests, I was good. Unfortunately, the truth was that while school had been easy for me, I lacked good study habits. I had to relearn how to study and manage my time.

So many Chicago people attended Grambling. We loved seeing each other make it down to Louisiana from the "crib"—that's what we called it. Whenever we needed a ride back home, we found people going back to the "crib." We had a club called the Windy City Club; Grambling had clubs for people from all over the world: The East Coast Club, The West Coast Club, and everything in between. I came to love Grambling, but it took a while for me to discover this love. I initially couldn't stand how slow and hot Louisiana was, but I didn't appreciate this until years later. I joined the Windy City Club and the National Association of Black Accountants. I met people from all over and made friends for life—people like I'Esha, Lolita, Mica, B, Puff, Jeff, and Kim, just to name a few. My childhood friend, Larry, was also there and his sister, Ramona, so that helped enormously to find familiar faces from the "crib" nearby when I needed a ride to the store or some food.

At Grambling, people walked or drove. There was only one franchise restaurant close to campus, Sonic; otherwise, we would have gone to the village or student union, besides the cafeteria, of course. They all close at a decent hour, so if you miss the time, you go hungry. I learned to appreciate the cafeteria after that first night without any money or food. I had a Snickers bar for dinner. I met a new guy in the cafeteria which sparked a relationship, to my surprise. But the fall semester of 1995 proved to be a struggle without a vehicle to get around. I hated depending on people to bring me somewhere. That is a hard adjustment coming from a big city. The "country" has no public transportation, no fleet of taxicabs, no 24-hour-open restaurants. I missed home quickly, especially the food. The weather was very different—super hot in Louisiana. The day usually started off cool, but by noon it was hot. I changed my clothes multiple times a day because of the heat.

Anthony and I broke up in January 1995. In March, that's when Mister came into the picture. He had been at Grambling for a year before I arrived, a psych major, born in Inglewood, California. But he also lived in Monroe, Louisiana, with his grandfather so he had a country accent. Mister cooked well, and that is the way to my heart. Here I was, hungry, poor, and dependent on others—particularly a man—for transportation and food. The hypocrisy of it all!

MAKING FAITH MOVES

The lessons I learned from my first year of college would get me through so many of life's struggles. I learned how to depend on myself. I maintained an open mind to learn about new cultures and speak up for myself. I learned how to circulate in a new environment and persevere. I celebrate my individuality; I longed to become a leader not a follower. I was determined to succeed by any means necessary to make myself and my family proud. I had come too far to turn back. I had to finish what I started, but I needed to find a way to buy what I needed to go away to college.

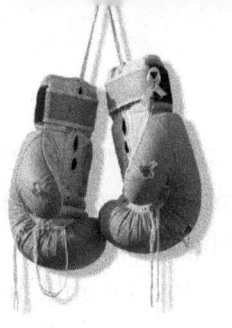

CHAPTER 10

Nikki Giovanni:
"MISTAKES ARE A FACT OF LIFE: IT IS THE RESPONSE TO THE ERROR THAT COUNTS."

During my first summer break from college, my father found me a job where he worked as a chef at the Hotel Intercontinental, as a hostess at their fine dining restaurant. Since my major was business management, specifically hotel/restaurant management before switching to accounting, working at the hotel gave me a bird's-eye view into hospitality management. Mister and I were still dating, even though I was home in Chicago for the summer and he was in Louisiana. We talked on the phone often and wrote each other letters all summer.

For the fall semester of 1995, once again I found a ride to college and took a full class load. My brother didn't return to college because his father signed him up for the U.S. Marines where he served our country for seventeen years.

Mister and I were together often off campus at his cousin Tasha's house, where he cooked for us all. I began smoking marijuana heavily around this time and enjoyed the freedom it brought to my mind. But this was horrible for my grades; I began procrastinating on projects and assignments. I spent the night off campus with no regard for getting a ride back for my classes. When my father called me first thing in the morning, I would be so tired from partying all night, although I still answered his calls. My girl, Esha, would tell me about going to class and trying to do better. Esha and I had begun hanging out more and getting to know each other since we both majored in accounting and came from the Windy City. Through Esha I met Lolita, Mica, Mike, Carmen, LaQuita, Danielle, and Vexton. This semester was not a highlight of my life: I ended it on academic probation. For that reason and because I really needed a car in college, I decided not to return after the fall semester. I took a break to go home, regroup, and work hard to purchase a car. I knew that if I didn't get it for myself, then I wouldn't have it at all.

In January 1996, I moved back home temporarily, and luckily my father found me that Hotel Inter-continental job. At that time, I reconnected with my friend from Hyde Park, Naishon, and discussed getting our own apartment together. She got a job at Hotel Inter-continental where I was working. I also enrolled in Harold Washington College two days a week, retaking some of the prerequisites that I did poorly on at Grambling previously. I worked five days a week at the Hotel and attended school full-time on my two off days. I had no days off; every day I got up early to catch the bus downtown for either work or school. Thankfully, my stepfather Larry occasionally lets me drive his car back and forth to school. Naishon and I agreed to be roommates at an apartment on 77th South Shore Drive. Since we both worked at the Hotel Inter-continental, it was a good arrangement for a while—at least. I maintained that for six months before I felt worn out. To be at work on time, I had to leave at 5:00 a.m. to catch two CTA buses. One day after working my 6:30 a.m. to 2:30 p.m. shift, I came home so exhausted that I fell asleep in my clothes. I woke up thinking it was the next day. I began running the shower and just so happened to turn on the Weather Channel when I noticed the date was still the same. I didn't even know the difference; I was so tired.

One night while I was at the bus stop on 67th Jeffrey, gunshots rang out. It was chaos. I watched a guy shooting in my direction as he ran across the street in the opposite direction. I froze until an older gentleman grabbed me and said, "Get down!" Thank God for angels among us. I was as frozen as the day I was asked by the creep at the cleaners to see my young breasts when I was 12 years old. I was so numb to violence by now that the idea of getting shot didn't even phase me. Once it was over, I waited for my bus to come as if nothing had happened. About ten years later I found myself in a carjacking situation while out in the city celebrating my birthday with my cousin Tee and our friend Tanya. Someone pulled a gun on her to take her car while we were sitting in it and fortunately, she took off accelerating down the street. My cousin Tee and I ducked down in the back seat just in case the guy starting shooting at us, there was no screams, shouts or words as Tanya drove us to safety.

Sharing an apartment with Naishon didn't really allow me to save money for a car as I had planned. I moved back with my mother and stepfather, quit school, and found a new job to get enough money so I could get that car and return to Grambling. I used the Career Resource Department at Harold Washington College to update my résumé and find a higher-paying job. I especially wanted to work only Monday through Friday so I could party with my friends on the weekends. I found Zonta International, a nonprofit organization advocating for women's rights, equality, education, and an end to child marriage and gender-based violence. At Zonta, I worked five days a week sitting at a nice desk, instead of running on my feet at a hotel all day. I was assigned to work in member services as a front-desk receptionist. Lanette was my manager at Zonta, and I really looked up to her. She was a Black woman who carried herself like a boss, ten years older than I. She lived up north, was a college graduate, and dressed nicely and classy. Thanks to this job, I saved enough to buy a 1991 sky-blue Pontiac Grand Am with tinted windows. My cousin Terry went with me to the dealership. I was so excited to have my own car at last. I drove all around the city that summer, partying with my friends Maxine, Shantea, Phenia, and Ganell.

The summer of 1996, my friends and I created a crew we named BOM. We all had BOM names, held cookouts at the beach, and moved as a unit all around the city but mostly on the Southside. My sister, my cousins, Shantea, Maxine, and Phenia. I loved hanging out with these ladies—no competition among us, no comparing, no backbiting, no drinking or smoking. Just positive vibes. I admired and respected them for how they all held down families with children and said exactly what they meant and meant what they said. They are all beautiful, inside and outside. Once I have a friend, their family becomes my family. We show up for each other. I can trust them with my money, my man, and my heart. I can trust them for their honesty, loyalty, and camaraderie. They accept me even when I am doing too much (my norm). I can shine as brightly as I want and don't need to dim my light around them—and vice versa.

Maxine would drop off my godson, Amirius, at my mom's house early in the morning when I was home from college. I looked after him and would take him to school while she went to work. She would randomly ask for help, trusting I would be there for her without question—and she was right. I used to buy him stuff, like his first pair of Jordan's. My first goddaughter told me I was her godmother because that's what she wanted. I fell in love with my Jalesa, who's always been my pretty girl. Jalesa is Shantea and Ganell's second daughter, and they did not object to her choice for godmother.

We hung out strong most weekends, going to clubs, trying out restaurants we could afford. When August rolled around, I was ready for Grambling with my new car. Two days before driving off, I went to the free clinic to check on my private parts—something I had begun doing since being raped. Rumor was spreading that the guy who raped me had AIDS. Thank goodness all my tests were negative for AIDS or HIV. I went to my friend Maxine's grandma's house to hang out before I left for school and told her my test for AIDS was negative. She pushed my shoulder to say, "Quit playing, girl, you know you aint got no AIDS." When she pushed me jokingly, my left foot twisted in my red Air Force Ones. I tried stepping on it but had to limp back to my car. I thought nothing more of it until that night when I went to bed. I had to elevate my foot on pillows because of the swelling. In the morning, I couldn't walk or stand on my left foot. I had to go to the doctor. I dressed and picked up Maxine so she could accompany me to the ER, especially as she had messed up my foot up. At Trinity Hospital ER, they determined I had broken my baby toe. They gave me an ugly shoe to wear and said it would heal in a month. I purchased a fly cane to help me walk instead of those horrible crutches and left for Grambling the next day.

I made the 12-hour drive alone. Luckily some good friends, Worm and Zeno, allowed me to stay with them in Grambling low-income housing for a semester while I worked at a law firm. I helped them pay the apartment bills. I wasn't enrolled in school that semester, but I enrolled the next. My friend Shay was looking for a roommate, and since I needed my own place, we decided to get an apartment in Ruston, the next town over from Grambling.

Mister and I spent Christmas in Chicago with my family. This was our first 12-hour road trip together. My family and friends liked him, so I was happy about that. We decided to spend the new year in Louisiana, so we had to time our trip to arrive there before midnight.

In January 1998, I enrolled full-time at Grambling, working on campus, and sharing an apartment with Shay. Two weeks into the new year, I found out I was pregnant. I had post-traumatic stress disorder (PTSD), always secretly fearing I couldn't get pregnant because I was raped. Thank God each time I went to the doctor, I tested negative for AIDS. However, in my first year in college, I had a foul odor and thick discharge from my vagina. I was so embarrassed; I didn't know what to do. It turned out I was not cleaning that area properly mainly due to the sexual abuse I had experienced, and no one taught me how. I didn't like to touch myself inside. I was so uncomfortable with my body—I had a love/hate relationship with it—mostly hate. I had no one, I felt comfortable enough to discuss these issues with my body. But I talked to God. I learned I could go to the infirmary on campus for health issues, and they said I had a bacterial infection. Thank God nothing worse.

Back in January 1998, when I was visiting my girl Tumeka in her dorm, I kept eating all her snacks, especially pickles. She said, *"You're greedy but not this greedy. You might be pregnant."* She rode with me to the store to purchase a pregnancy test, and I took it back to her dorm. It was positive for pregnancy. I was shocked but not surprised. I had always said I didn't want to *ever* get married or have children. I just wanted to be wealthy and travel this world as a lawyer. On one hand, I felt happy that I could get pregnant after the rape. But then reality hit: I was a broke college student trying to graduate and had no stability.

I went to the housing department to apply for low-income housing and/or Section 8 housing in anticipation of being a mother. I included that I was pregnant in my application and looking for a two-bedroom. They said they would contact me when my name came up on the waiting list to receive my voucher. I made a doctor's appointment at the local free clinic in Ruston, where Shay and I lived. My results indicated I was six weeks pregnant. I applied for food stamps and Medicaid. I needed time to process before sharing this news with my family or Mister. I started working harder in my classes because I now had another person depending on my success. I also had to recover from being on academic probation during the semester I left school. I had a 1.9 GPA, the result of hanging out, smoking weed, and not studying. But I redeemed myself in the spring of 1998, earning great grades and making the dean's list for the first time.

The baby turned out to be identical twin boys who were born at 26 weeks after I was in labor for seven days. I moved back home after giving birth during my summer break in 1998.

MAKING FAITH MOVES

Having to leave Grambling to go back home twice made me feel like a failure, but I knew I had a plan. I was holding on to faith no matter what. I read somewhere that regret looks back, and frustration looks around, but faith looks forward. Faith fixes our gaze on God's promises and moves us ahead in anticipation and hope. I was hopeful. When I received my poor grades and was on academic probation, I was disappointed in myself and vowed not to let that happen again. I began thinking about my future and if I wanted to begin the life I always wanted, it was up to me to make it good. I couldn't go back home and live with my mother or father forever. I couldn't blame my lack of achievement on anyone but myself. I was determined to succeed and had a plan. I slowed down partying, stopped smoking weed, and stopped all alcohol. I believed one must sacrifice if one wants a change in life. So, I sacrificed partying for the life I was after. I mean, what would Claire Huxtable do? I learned my lessons from failure; mistakes are a part of life; it matters how you address and abound from them.

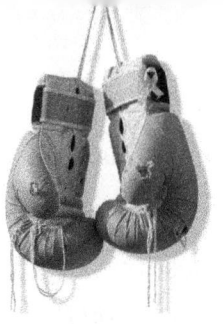

CHAPTER 11

Jay L:
"EVERYBODY CAN TELL YOU HOW TO DO IT, BUT THEY NEVER DONE IT."

A month after the twins turned one year old, I was at work in Chicago at Zonta International, and a new position opened which would be a promotion opportunity for me. I applied and spoke to the director about the opening. The director, Janet, told me that job was going to Pam, but she wanted me to train her. I asked why Pam would get the job over me when I already knew the job well. Janet explained because Pam had a bachelor's degree in liberal arts, and I didn't have my bachelor's in accounting yet. I fumed at my desk after that conversation. I called my favorite accounting professor, Dr. Cunningham, and told him about my frustrations. He asked about school, and I told him how many credits would transfer from Grambling to Chicago State.

"Well, come back to Grambling," he said.

Me: "I have twins now. What about housing, and daycare?"

Dr. Cunningham: "Cassandra, just come back to Grambling, you can get family housing, I can put your classes in the system *now, you don't have that much time before you graduate. We'll help you figure it out."*

I couldn't think of any questions that he couldn't answer. I wrote my two-week letter of resignation that day. I hated that Zonta told me "No" for any position, especially one I knew I could do well. So, my mind was set to finish Grambling and get my degree.

That evening, I told Mister about going back to school. We began thinking about where to stay and how much it would cost. His family lived in Monroe, thirty minutes from the school. My great-grandmother, who used to babysit and absolutely loved those babies, was upset when I told her I was going back to school in Louisiana. *"You are not taking these babies,"* she told me. I said, *"Grandma, they must go with me, they are my babies!"* I loved her for wanting to keep my babies—she was one of the few people I could trust to keep them without question or complaint. But still...

Mister's aunt Carrie loaned us the money for the U-Haul and gas back to Louisiana. I found someone to take over our apartment lease. Mister drove the U-Haul, and I followed him in the Buick Skylark with our 1-year-old twin sons for our 12-hour road trip. I called Grambling Housing prior to coming down, and they confirmed my name was at the top of the waiting list for a two-bedroom for me and my baby. I now informed them that now I had twins, but they said I still only qualified for a two-bedroom. They were babies and could share a room.

The twins and I stayed with my friends Esha and Vex at their two-bedroom apartment for a couple of weeks waiting on my Section 8 voucher from Grambling. Esha and Vex were so welcoming, and I'm forever indebted to them for allowing us to live with them until we found our own place. I called around and decided to select the two-bedroom/two-bath furnished apartment closest to the university just in case my car broke down, so I could still get to classes.

I thought of anything and everything: I got approved for Medicaid, food stamps, WIC, and childcare vouchers. One of my professors, Dr. Nwokoma, mentioned he and his wife operated childcare from their home and would take very good care of my babies. I set it up with the childcare vouchers. Two of my friends, Shon and E, also had baby boys and we worked out a system to drop off and pick up our babies five days a week. Shon was married to my friend Pac, and they also had an older baby girl named Mariah. I did work-study on campus, attended classes full-time, and took care of my twins. Due to their developmental delays, they were behind other babies their same age. But I didn't worry because I knew they were strong—I saw how they fought as preemies. I was just grateful God heard my cries of making sure they survived, after the dire news the doctor told me.

After we settled into our apartment, with schedules intact and budget set, my friend Tumeka called to say she was coming back to school with her baby girl and wanted to stay with me until she got on her feet. I agreed and said sure, I made room for them in the twins' room. Tumeka didn't have a car, so I let her use mine from time to time if she needed, the way Esha and Vex had done for me and my babies. Whenever anyone stayed with me, I never charged them because I understood people needed to save their money to live on their own.

My best friends, Maxine and Shantea, called me about a great concert coming to Chicago—the How High tour with Method Man, Redman, Jay Z, and DMX. I was a huge fan of them all, especially Jay and DMX, so I told them to buy a ticket, and I would pay them back. I decided to leave my twins at home with Mister and Tumeka, so I wouldn't have to take them for a weekend trip. Tumeka later told me that Mister made advances towards her. When I confronted him, he said she came on to him. But I did nothing again. Years later, I learned Mister made advances towards someone else while staying in my apartment when I was in class.

Eventually, Tumeka and her baby girl went back home to the DMV area because for some reason she couldn't get enrolled in school. Mister's cousin, Chelle, came down from Monroe with her daughter, Destiny, who was the same age as my twins. Mister took the car and disappeared the whole weekend in Monroe or wherever and returned late Sunday night so I could go to school and work on Monday. I said nothing. I had no capacity to monitor his movements. I'm sure it presented itself as being nonchalant, but it was my defense mechanism to protect my heart.

Mister's niece moved down to Grambling from California because his older sister was having problems with her young teenage daughter and wanted her to get out of California for a while. She lived with his sister's best friend who lived near us in Grambling. I used to drop his niece off at school and pick her up. We were there to support her and make sure she was safe and loved.

My classes were predominantly in the Business College at this time, and I completed most of my prerequisites for my accounting major. I was involved in or led class projects, and I organized study groups in between parenting and working. My schedule was very tightly coordinated, and time management was a priority because I couldn't afford to fail. I was on my third attempt at completing the requirements for my bachelor's degree. I was in survival mode, and so exhaustion, frustration, and disconnection became my new norm. I honestly don't know how I managed to be a mother to my twins during this time on auto pilot. I had come so far but it still felt so distant to graduate. When my car needed repairs, I had to find a solution. My friend Pac usually came through for me and my twins with a reliable mechanic I could afford who wouldn't take advantage of me.

My twins were making great strides in their development by being around Dr. Nwokoma's large family. They were a tremendous help to me as a new mom, and I learned so much from them. The twins' personalities were emerging each day. Deon was a natural-born leader who led with his head. He was very strong-willed and used to antagonize Neon enough until Neon started fighting back. Neon was naturally very loving and led with his heart; he was caring and selfless. Together, they were the cutest babies, full of happiness and joy. I dressed them alike every day in the most adorable outfits, and they were the talk of the campus whenever I took them out. People often remarked I should get them on television because they were identical twins. They both fiercely protected each other even from me. On more than one occasion I might discipline one of them, but the other would defend his brother by yelling at me in baby language and hitting me back. I loved how they protected one another, and I advocated for that throughout their lives to always take care of one another, no matter what. Every decision I made included consideration of what was best for them and their futures. They were my motivation to finish what I started, to be the best version of me.

I made two new friends around this time: Nikki and Crystal. Crystal was from the west side of Chicago—I met her through Esha; Nikki from Elgin, Illinois, was the girlfriend of my friend Larry; they had two little girls. As a young mother too, Nikki could relate to my struggles. We had many playdates with my twins and her sweet little girls.

My first semester back in school was very difficult, but I made the dean's list with my full schedule. I was determined to bring my GPA up before graduating to put myself in a better competitive situation. I made my class schedule for the next semester, Spring of 2000, in December 1999. Each day, I worked hard toward my purpose of graduating.

Mister and I took the twins home for Christmas to Chicago to stay at my mom and stepfather's house. As usual when I visited home, I went to my Aunt Sharon and Uncle Jobe house to pick up my cousin Karen, and we got our hair done either from Paulette or Toya and shopped at the Ford City mall. Karen had graduated from Dunbar High School, class of 1999, so she was excited about starting college in January. I partied with my BOM friends at nightclubs and restaurants all over Chicago. My sister Maxine's mother, Francine, gave me the nickname, "Get It done Sandy" because she said I always got the job done. I saw most of my family and friends while visiting home at Christmas and drove back to school after New Year's Day.

MAKING FAITH MOVES

On Sundays, we attended church service for fellowship at Zion Traveler Baptist church. My relationship with God was by far my strongest relationship. I recited this scripture daily: Phil 4:13: I can do all things through Christ. It strengthened me through many days and nights. When I was away in college after purchasing my car, I traveled 12 hours by myself many times between Chicago and Grambling. At times on my driving journey, I encountered storms, and had to slow down, turn up my windshield wipers, and move closer to my windshield to see better. I noticed many cars stopped under a bridge until the rain diminished. But I never stopped. I kept going because I knew eventually the storm would end and I didn't want to waste time waiting. Storms don't last. When I pray and I encounter such a particularly tough time that it feels like I am scaling a mountain, I don't ask God to move the mountain. Instead, I ask God for the strength to climb it.

Matthew 17:20 KJV: And Jesus said unto them, Because of your unbelief: for verily I say unto you, if ye have faith as a grain of mustard seed, ye shall say unto this mountain, remove hence to yonder place; and it shall remove; and nothing shall be impossible unto you.

I was blazing my own trail, and that is not easy to do when you have no precedent for it. Before me, I didn't see anyone who moved between home to college while raising two special babies. Of course, many had accomplished such a thing before. I clung to my imaginations of those pioneers. My ancestors endured harsh conditions to progress our people, and I stand on their shoulders. This vision kept me forging ahead when I wanted to stop. I chose not to be influenced by individuals attempting to instruct me on matters with which they had no personal experience.

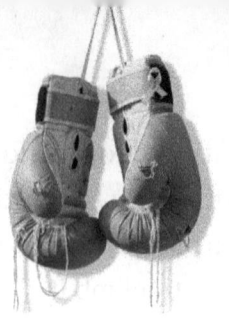

CHAPTER 12

Langston Hughes: "THE ONLY WAY TO GET A THING DONE IS TO START TO DO IT, THEN KEEP ON DOING IT, AND FINALLY YOU'LL FINISH IT."

Classes in the spring of 2000 classes. I had mostly accounting classes which I loved, since I was moving into my major more directly. I could now determine how I would use my accounting degree in my future career.

At the end of January, my babies caught cold. They had asthma and were breathing harder, so I took them to the ER. I hated seeing my babies sick. Being in the hospital with them triggered my memories of their birth and stay in the NICU. They were put in crib beds surrounded by plastic like a huge nebulizer treatment. I asked the doctor what I could do to help with their asthma. He advised I not smoke around them. Since I didn't, that was no problem—but Mister did. I created a new rule right away: No smoking around my babies. We were so happy to go back home after three days in the hospital. The twins got their own nebulizer and asthma pump.

As I began unpacking our hospital bags, I received a phone call and heard a sound I will never forget. My father was crying as he told me my cousin Karen had died from an asthma attack. From that moment until God knows when, I was in auto pilot survivor mode, broken-hearted and never to be the same. Here, I had literally returned from the twins' hospital stay because of asthma, and now I am learning that my first cousin, my best friend and little sister, had died from something similar. We later found out she had a blood clot in her lungs. I was beyond agony. It seemed that everything worked against me while I was trying to get my degree. I felt defeated. It was too much: I was almost six years out of high school, twice a college dropout, mother to twins, a thousand miles away from home, and now an unbearable loss. Lord, have mercy.

I told Mister what happened and said we had to go back to Chicago. I couldn't think about packing a suitcase. I grabbed dirty laundry bags and cleaned clothes and threw them in the car along with any other necessity. I was in a trance, but I knew I needed to get home immediately. Mister and I were just not in a good place in our relationship, but I needed him to help me drive and keep the boys while I did what my family needed me to do. We encountered an ice storm on the highway through Arkansas. We had to pull over because we were too fatigued to drive through the night, and we couldn't afford a hotel. We slept a few hours in the car bundled up with the twins, then got back on the road to Chicago.

I cannot recall the days, hours, or minutes of this trip. I don't recall who I visited or who visited me. I knew my Auntie Sharon asked me to pick an outfit for Karen's burial because Karen and I often shopped together. I found myself, numb, trance-like, at Karen's funeral. Seeing her lying in that coffin messed me up. She was too young, too beautiful, too good...January 29, 2000, the day that messed me up.

I went back to school severely depressed. I was merely existing. I could not be bothered with my relationship with Mister. I could only focus on the twins' well-being and getting my degree so I could take better care of us. I had to have tunnel vision. I lost weight on my already small-framed body. My friends Lolita and Esha had graduated already, but I still had two semesters to go.

My relationship with Mister was so on and off that I just blurted out we should end it. He could not console me of anything. When I made friends in my classes, Mister found out I was spending my time with a particular guy. He started arguing with me. We had a scuffle in our bedroom. He grabbed me by the collar of my t-shirt, which caused a scratch my neck. I pushed him away and he flew over the bed and fell to the other side. He seized my car keys and stormed out.

My cousin Karen had been gone only a month at this point, but I was emotionally drained and unhinged. I could not maintain this relationship anymore. Then one day, in my business management class, someone caught my attention. It was a nice distraction.

Enter Brick City! His swagger, his intelligence, his smile, his skin. He walked around with an air of not being impressed by anyone. He wasn't trying to fit in. He did whatever felt right for him, and that included how he expressed his style in dress. I began flirting with him with my eyes until he approached me to ask if I knew how to braid hair. I said yeah, lying my butt off (I could braid hair about as good as I could cook—which was not at all—but I said whatever got me close to this dude.) Those braids were so bogus, and I was so embarrassed, but it was my excuse to get to know him. No one had caught my attention in years. We cover all kinds of topics, from music to geography. His intelligence was so refreshing. I had never met someone my age who had visited Africa. His perspective was intriguing, and I admired him for that. We hung out after class, and it was like breathing fresh air again. I am attracted to intelligence and ambition.

He called me beautiful every day, showing me so much tenderness. He would play the Dru Hill song, "Beauty" for me and express how he felt being with me. At a time, all I saw was men wanting a woman who is ride or die for them. They were expecting performative resilience in their women for their love, possibly including their loyalty, a woman willing to ride or die for/with them, through infidelity, drama and abuse. Brick City didn't ask anything of my love, he just wanted its presence in his life. I will never forget one day we were hanging out at my apartment and his roommate DC called to see if he wanted to go hoop. I heard him say, "*Hold on, let me check to see if it's cool with my Queen.*" YO! A man checking with his woman before making plans with his friends—I had never heard of it. I was turned on, seen, honored. I felt like it mattered to him what I wanted. Most men I knew was all about "bros before hoes," so this level of maturity was unique. Consequently, when he asked me if we had any plans today because his boys wanted to play basketball, I told him to go and have fun! This was most of our relationship, him working at a high emotional intelligence and me acting like an unhealed baby girl.

Brick City offered to pick up my boys after his classes to give me a break some days. He knew I was struggling since Karen's death. He made us playdates at the park with my boys. He began planning that we would marry, and our honeymoon would be in Egypt where they had black sand beaches. I had never had a conversation with a man planning out our wedding to me or talking about foreign lands. We dated for about nine months, during which he graduated from Grambling, I met his family, I visited Newark, and he visited

Chicago. But when I went back to school in the fall, he wasn't with me, and I ended it with him because Mister asked for us to get back together. Brick City taught me so much about myself—about a man who could love, respect, and trust how I desired to be treated and that it is possible to have a healthy relationship. I didn't have to be a hard rock because, in his eyes, I was a gem. He recognized the queen in me and treated me as such.

Chicago raised me tough. I kept a tough exterior and nonchalant attitude in relationships that certainly came across as heartless, but it was my way of protecting myself from ever losing control again. In my mind, being out of control got me raped. Brick City constantly challenged that about me and added more love to my meanness. When I went back to school in fall 2000, Mister called and immediately came back to Grambling to visit the twins. I had not heard from him all summer; he never called to check on the twins, but here he was now! He helped me settle back in, cleaned my apartment while I bathed the twins before bed. Eventually we reunited, and I called Brick City to break up with him. That was the hardest thing I ever did. Breaking his heart broke my heart too. I had never felt that way. My excuse was "I hurt you before you hurt me"—an act I learned after being raped at 16. But I knew I owed Brick City an honest conversation about my decision to end our relationship. Walking away from love like that hurt me, and for the first time, I felt compassion for a man outside of my family.

Immediately after breaking off with Brick City, I regretted it. Mister took my boys to visit his family in Monroe, giving me some alone time for a few days. When I went to pick them up, Mister was at his cousin's house with other family members, including our babies, and in bed with his cousin's neighbor! The family saw me pulling up, so by the time I entered, she was leaving through a back room and cussing him out as she left. Of course, I lamented leaving Brick City to put up with this foolishness.

My only understanding was that I wanted my twins to have a relationship with their father, and that implied I had to be with him too. I was raised my entire life with my father and my mother and knew how important that was to a child. So, I felt that regardless of my needs, my sons needed their father. So, I adjusted my emotions, settled for less, and played the role of staying with him. Personally, I concentrated on raising my twins and getting my degree. My heart was still raw from missing my cousin Karen; her first birthday since she passed was approaching September 17th, and I was in pain. I couldn't really manage my relationship with Mister. We were together, but he came and went as he pleased, and I couldn't afford to care. Mister never asked about my classes or progress, and I never asked him about his whereabouts. I knew I couldn't depend on him, so I didn't. I made sure I earned enough money to cover the rent, car note, gas, food, utilities, books, childcare, and so on, and he chipped in when/if he was working. And that was our relationship, from beginning to end.

I had been on a roll with my grades since returning to school with my new car in 1997. After I lost my cousin Karen in the spring 2000 semester, I fell off the dean's list, so I knew I had to work even harder the next two semesters to graduate in the class of 2001 with an average GPA. I knew this semester had so much on the line, and I needed to set up an internship. I researched companies to work in and school where I could pick up a master's immediately after graduating.

I was also helping my babies reach their developmental milestones. Thankfully, they had no more asthma issues. They were my source of joy and inspiration but also my fears about being a good mother for them. My main promise was I would always be present in their lives.

The fall semester, I managed to excel in my grades and appear again on the dean's list. As I registered for spring, I noted that if I took seven courses, I could finish with one class in the summer. To take seven classes (21 credit hours!), I had to get approval from the department head. I remember pleading with Dr. Wilkerson, the head of the Accounting Department, to sign off. He was concerned that the load of all senior level accounting courses would be too much with my twins plus work-study. I assured him I was willing to put in the work. Finally convinced, he approved. I don't know when or if I slept at all that semester, but I crushed it in my classes—all A's in seven courses.

The U.S. Department of Treasury came to one of my senior-level accounting courses to discuss careers and let us know they were here for our job fair. I prepared my résumé and donned my best navy-blue pants suit. I had recently come back from visiting home for the weekend and got my hair done by Paulette, my friend and stylist, since I was 16. I add that in here because the representative from the U.S. government said she remembered me because she loved how my hair was cut in layers and looked nice and healthy. She began telling me about the division she worked in, which was the criminal investigation division. I remember their claim to fame was bringing down Al Capone. She informed me of the duties required to be a special agent for the U.S. Department of Treasury, one of which would require physical training for six months away from my children. That didn't fit me as a mother of two-year-old twins. However, she mentioned other more suitable careers and forwarded my application to another division. They contacted me to come in for an interview in June 2001; I let them know my graduation date was July 13, 2001, and we scheduled my interview for five days after my graduation—on my mother's birthday no less, July 18, 2001. The interview was in Cincinnati, and I had to pack up before graduation to drive from Louisiana to Chicago and then to Cincinnati. God was certainly working it out!

My college graduation was a day of complete joy, although my heart still ached that Karen couldn't be there. This was a dream realized from a dream deferred for seven years. Still without much money, I made my own invitations and mailed them to family and friends. My twins were three years old now, and they were in the audience, able to see their mother walking across the stage. My parents, stepparents, stepsister, cousins Marcus, Tinesha, and Aireale, and Aunt Bettye came to support me. They drove down from Chicago, their first visit to Grambling. Unise and her baby boy Demetrius got on the Greyhound bus from Chicago to attend. My sister, Jeanette, drove from North Carolina with my nephews. My friends Erika, Shon, Pac, Esha, and Vex were all there as well.

My graduation day was a beautiful, sunshiny day at the auditorium on the Grambling State University campus. I wore a brown and tan knee-length wrap-dress with a modest stiletto heel. I dressed my twins in Baby Gap matching outfits with bucket hats. I left the house first since I had to be there early to line up, and I didn't know where my family would be sitting but I heard my babies crying in the audience. When my name was called, I wanted to stand on that stage in that special moment for a while. I stood tall, honoring my ancestors before me, my family and friends now with me, and my legacy forever more as a college graduate. I promised myself to finish my goal. I had overcome so much, and victory was mine. This girl from the Southside of Chicago turned woman and mother had achieved a miraculous feat. "Sandy got it done," just like Mrs. Francine said. She saw me before I did.

After graduation, Mister barbecued, and some of my friends—Ericka, Esha, Vex, Fred, Shon and Pac—stopped by my apartment to celebrate. Although I didn't drink, I felt okay to toast one with my family and friends.

MAKING FAITH MOVES

I think back on my audacity to leave home at 18, with no money, no transportation, no idea of living on my own. I had a dream of graduating from college so I could provide a better life myself, my family and my community. As Phil 4:13 reads, I had faith that I can do all things through Christ which strengthens me. Through trial and error, starts and stops, disappointments and grief, I graduated from Grambling State University with my Bachelor of Science degree as an accounting major on July 13, 2001. I wanted to live in that moment and absorb all its feelings. I was a college graduate, and nobody could take that away from me! It took me seven years, with a set of three-year-old twin sons, but thank God, I made it. I never gave up on myself. Keep believing in yourself. God put a dream inside of you because that is who you are. Envision your future self-doing whatever is in you to do. Prioritize personal growth, make necessary sacrifices for long-term benefits, and maintain consistent discipline.

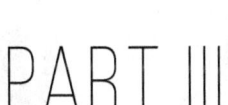

PART III

THE CANCER—WHAT DOESN'T KILL YOU MAKES YOU STRONGER

For I know the plans I have for you, declares the Lord, plans to prosper you and not to harm you, plans to give you hope and a future. (Jeremiah 29:11)

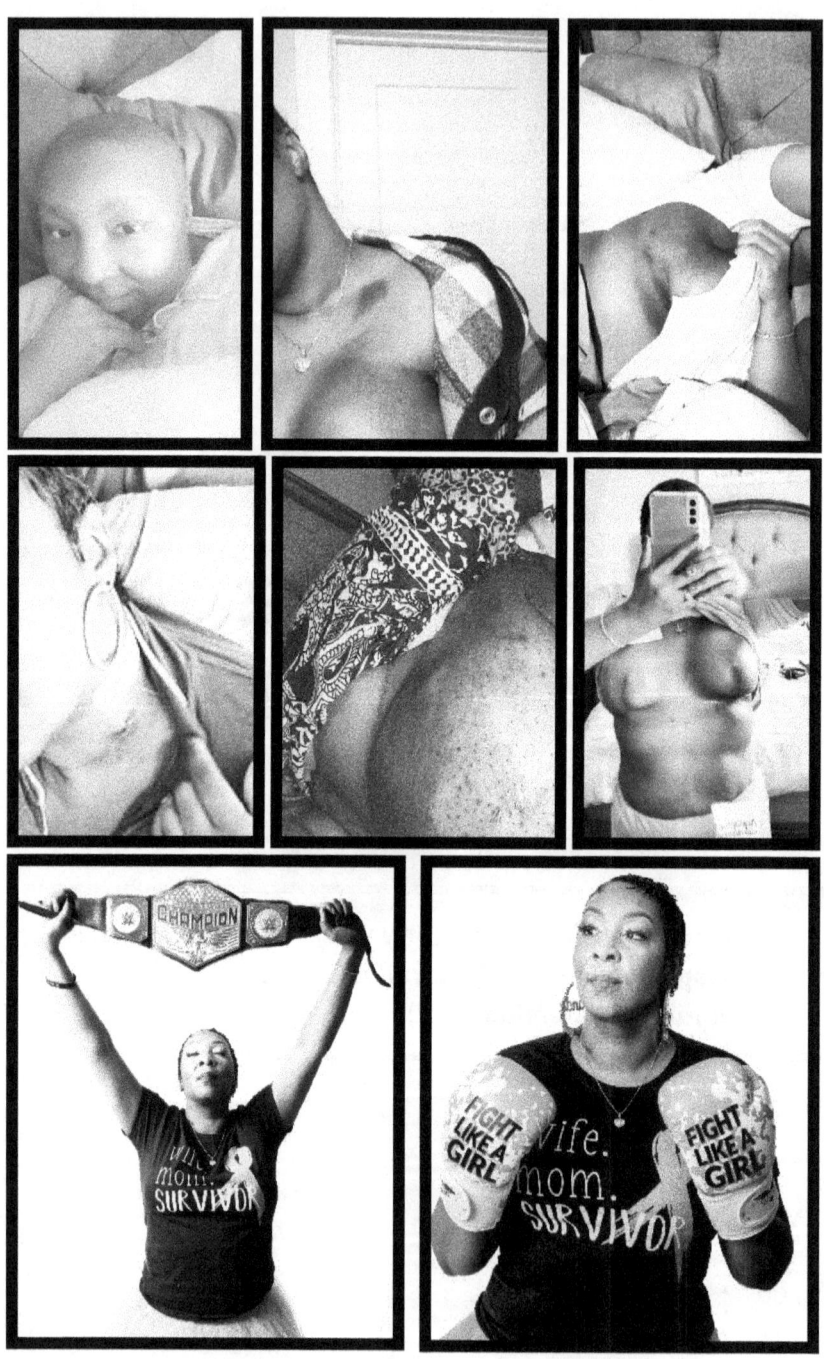

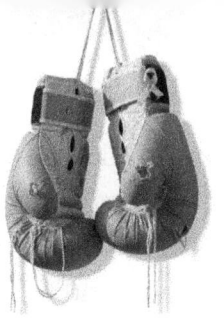

CHAPTER 13

James Baldwin: "LOVE IS A BATTLE; LOVE IS A WAR; LOVE IS A GROWING UP."

One of the main reasons my culture celebrates Black love so viciously is because it had been a point of contention since my ancestors were kidnapped from their homeland to come to the United States of America. There have always been systems put in place to separate the black man from the black woman. The Masters (Massas) of the enslaved would sell Black men to other plantation owners away from the plantation where they worked with their wives and children, leaving the Black women and children to fend for and protect themselves. Massa would rape the enslaved women, girls, and even boys. Massa would impregnant these women and girls but never claim their babies, which made them the original deadbeat Daddies. This is also one reason Black Americans come in so many different hues.

This practice continued through the centuries. In the 1970s, if women needed public assistance known as welfare, they were granted it if no man was living in the home with them. So, women would hide or leave the man to take financial care of themselves and their children. It was widely known that you could not have a man in your home and get welfare assistance. This caused separations once again between Black men and women.

There is a myth that Black families are missing their fathers; however, the conversation is omitting the fact that Black men have been falsely imprisoned, killed, lynched, and murdered by such groups like the Ku Klux Klan (KKK), FBI, CIA, and police. Dr. Martin Luther King and Malcolm X were both assassinated and under surveillance by the FBI. The KKK, founded in 1865, has murdered men and women throughout our history simply because of their race, nationality, religion, or lifestyle. The KKK ideology is anti-Black racism, white supremacy, white nationalism. Unlike the Black Panthers whom the FBI targeted and murdered until they no longer exist, the KKK still exists to this day under different names and job titles.

The FBI had a counterintelligence program (cointelpro) which was used to sabotage through legal force the Black Panthers, and in December 1969, the FBI along with the Chicago Police Department raided and assassinated local Black Panther party leader Fred Hampton and other Black Panthers. I read Assata Shakur's book on the abuse and devastation that the Black Panthers experienced while advocating for Black Americans. It served as a reminder of the discrimination encountered based on skin color specifically targeting black men.

Another factor that contributed to the disruption of Black families was the impact of drugs. For about a decade, a San Francisco drug ring sold cocaine to the Black gang leaders of Los Angeles, which then funneled millions in drug money to a Latin America army run by the CIA. Many Black individuals became involved with drugs in various ways—as sellers, users, or through addiction to both drugs and the financial gains from selling them. Subsequently, numerous people were arrested and imprisoned for extended periods, resulting in significant impacts on their families and communities. This was by design, the government in charge of bringing it to our community knew exactly what would happen. The sale of drugs was depicted as a means of generating income to support families. However, the black people involved in drug distribution often did not consider the significant impact this activity would have on communities, including long-term consequences such as addiction, family disruption, and increased incarceration rates across generations. The television series, Snowfall, by John Singleton, depicts this perfectly. Police forces have been exposed as selling crack cocaine to inner-city communities, getting paid for it, and then locking up the drug dealers once they were paid in full by the drug dealers.

American policing is a huge factor in the destruction of the black family and systematic racism. Slave patrols were armed groups of men down South who policed slaves, especially those labeled as defiant. Slave patrols were the first unofficial police in America with one mission: to establish a system of terror and stop slave uprisings. They are considered an early form of American policing. American policing can lead to death for Black people.

Rest in peace and love, my brothers and sisters: Amadou Diallo, Eric Garner, Laquan McDonald, Michael Brown, Sean Bell, Botham Jean, Sandra Bland, Breonna Taylor, Eugene Pitchford, Jimmie Lee Jackson, Tamir Rice, Daunte Wright, and respectfully countless others who were unarmed and murdered by police. Honorable mention to Trayvon Martin who was a 17-year-old young man walking home from the store with Skittles and sweet tea and was murdered by a self-proclaimed safety officer I refuse to name who was acquitted of all charges. The false narratives that try to blame Black-on-Black crime for the decline of our race is no more real than white-on-white crime or any other race experiencing crime in their midst. Directly or indirectly, violence is often glorified and perceived as an essential part of Black culture. The idea of Black-on-Black crime is a myth because much of all violent crime in the United States happens between people of the same race. According to the Vera Institute of Justice, 57% of reported violent crimes committed against white victims were perpetrated by white offenders.

From the transatlantic slave trade, Jim crow, voting rights, civil rights, red lining, white flight, blue code of silence and the Tuskegee Syphilis Study just to name a few, we keep going!

When people design systems to defeat you, it means you are treasured and powerful. The enemy would not attack you if you did not have something valuable inside of you. As the saying goes, thieves don't break into empty houses. You have value. There is something worthy in each of us.

An African proverb says, if you want to go fast, go alone. If you want to go far, go together. I was done going fast, I wanted to go far.

If Black men and women can persevere through adversity and remain united despite obstacles and systems intended to keep us apart, that's strength—that's Black love.

The brilliant Nikki Giovanni said, Black love is Black wealth.

December 2014...Meeting my Forever.

I'm a movement by myself, but a force when we're together.

Joe and I met through an online dating website called Plenty of Fish. Online dating platforms continue to be viewed differently by various people. It is sometimes assumed that individuals who use these websites are unable to find partners independently, leading them to try online options. Joe and I are both individuals who have not encountered difficulties in finding potential partners, this time we were seeking deeper, more meaningful connections. I honestly don't know how we would have met otherwise, even though we later discovered we traveled in similar circles in similar areas of Chicago growing up. My schedule was my boys, working, church, home, family, and friends. I had a full life except for a partner. I was still running, always busy raising my children and working on my career. The twins were in high school and needed more of my time to keep them focused. After my last relationship, I completely considered not dating anyone until my youngest Son-shine, Zion, reached 18 years old. At this time, he was 8. I dated some great guys here and there, but nothing serious. Thus, when my cousin Aireale suggested a dating site for me, I highly objected and rejected the idea. She explained her logic: What did I have to lose? I obliged her so I could say at least say I tried.

We didn't find each other right away. I was on the site for eight months before we met. Joe sent me a message on the dating site to let me know he was interested and asked for my number. We went back and forward texting a couple times before he asked to have a conversation. Our initial conversation took place in December 2014, during the Christmas season. Drawing upon my experience as a former auditor, I applied effective interview techniques to facilitate a productive dialogue. I asked him probing questions about his upbringing, role models, music playlist, handling adversity (mentally, physically, spiritually), what happened to his last relationship (checking to see if he led with blaming the other person or was accountable for his choices), how long was his longest relationship (checking for commitment issues), did he have children and how many. I asked when he last cried and what caused it. He shared stories with me about his heartaches, pains, and downfalls. He shared how he had fought through depression and persevered. We stayed on the phone for over four hours. In that first conversation, he had me hooked. I wasn't interested in any materialistic items he accrued; I was more interested in the fabric of the man he was and his character after all, money don't make a man, a man makes the money. I needed to know he had a heart and was willing to share it. I wanted to know by the questions I asked about his relationship with God instead of where he attended church, I wanted to know how he leads, if he had intelligence. Titles did not matter to me, but his integrity did. He let me know he didn't have a car, was new at his job, and was currently staying with his mom. We agreed to meet up for the first time on December 22, 2014, at a local pub. I had just gotten my hair done, ran a few errands, threw on a cute pair of jeans and comfy blouse, and met him. He didn't have a car, so I picked him up at his mother's house. He approached with a nice physique, a handsome face, stylish clothes, a pleasant scent, and a nice smile. The conversations matched his energy. We vibed instantly.

We played pool on our second date. Our third date was New Year's Eve, December 31, 2014, at Sugarplum's (Aireale) party. We brought in the new year of 2015 together and have been together ever since. We loved spending time together while dating, enjoying each other's company and mutual attraction. Because I believed in him so much, I drove him to and from work every day for about a year until he purchased a car.

When we met, his daughter, JaNiya, was 10 years and his son, Joseph (I nicknamed him Jojo), was 3; I, of course, had three boys who were now 16 and 8. We blended our family of four boys and one girl and made sure each of them knew we were together and working on a permanent future. We supported their academic goals and extracurricular activities. Blending families is hard work because of the outside factors, however, the end goal and objective must always be the best interest of the children. We both wanted to raise good people, love and support them, and make sure they were healthy and happy. I advocate for children having a childhood free from having to become responsible adults too early in their lives.

Having managed independently for an extended period, I anticipated potential challenges in adjusting to the presence of another individual assuming household leadership. I never had to answer to anyone but God about the affairs of my children or how I ran my household. I didn't have to consider anyone else when I made decisions in the past concerning their lives. I now had to release control, trust a man to be who he says he is, and do what it takes to run our family. I know I am an Alpha female—a leader, strong and powerful. I believed I could create the life I wanted to live on my own, and now I realized that thinking had to change. I allowed my mindset, my actions, and my leadership style to be critiqued and changed to include Joe as the head of household. I now had someone to be accountable to, and vice versa.

Joe stepped in and made his presence as the head of the household known from the beginning by establishing a household budget and paying bills I used the word "I" a lot, and Joe pointed it out to me that we had to start using "we" because we are a team, and I was no longer doing everything by myself. Lord knows I was ready to take my Superwoman cape off and allow Joe to lead. One of our biggest issues is my independence, I battle with asking for help. I prefer someone help when I struggle.

When it came to being a stepmother, I knew my place in their lives. I took the role of being supportive and loving as a bonus parent, never to compete with their mothers. They carried those babies in their bodies; I carry them in my heart. I made sure to support each member of our family individually and together as a family unit. They were all great children with good hearts, and I loved them all as I love myself. JaNiya was to herself like Zion and me. Jojo was a lot like the twins and Joe, loving to play and watch sports. After mentoring so many girls and having goddaughters, I finally had a daughter to pour into right at home. I got to know both children and let them know they can always talk to me about anything. I wanted them to feel the same love I gave my Son-shines. I shared my space, my heart, my family, and my friends with them, and Joe did the same for my boys. We created a blended family filled with love.

Joe always took me out on dates, and I loved the way he held my hand and protected me. He made me feel safe when I was with him. He protected my peace. We went on trips out of town for birthdays and "just because." Our first big argument followed my old dating pattern. Someone would do something to make me mad, and I would rebel, walk away, ignore and ghost them until they begged me back, but no way would I contact them first, ever. I could give a person silent treatment forever. That changed with Joe. I missed him, and that's when I knew this was different. I needed to pay attention before I lost something special. I complained to my friends Ketari and Angel about him, and they would let me know if I was tripping or wrong. Which was usually the case. I admit I was a spoiled daddy's girl and was extra hard on men. I could not treat Joe this way. He made me communicate more and better, and we both determined we were worth fighting for.

We helped each other be our best selves as parents, as individuals, and as a couple. He held me accountable and checked me on my BS and I did the same for him. We realized it's better to listen and understand each other, rather than try to win an argument since we are on the same team.

We discussed our children's future, how we planned to support them, and what our financial health and goals were.

I decided to finally complete the requirements to achieve my MBA and return to school at Indiana Wesleyan University in 2017. Joe supported me by picking up my slack with the children and purchasing a new laptop for me to complete my studies online. He worked on building my credit report—I never had anyone this invested in making sure I had good credit! Once our credit scores were higher, we had plans on buying a house together. We liked our area and wanted Zion to remain in his school district, so we determined the area for purchase. This was also new territory for me since I purchased my first home by myself when I was 31. Working a full-time job, going house hunting, growing in my relationship, being a full-time parent and a full-time student was a lot to achieve.

I love learning and I am always up for a great challenge. It took me a year in a half to attend classes online daily after work, studying executive leadership and global management. We finally found a house we both loved and purchased it together on April 1, 2018. I graduated with my Master of Business Administration degree in April 2019. My children, parents, brother, sister, and nieces were all there to witness me walking across another stage. Joe showered me with so many gifts, decorated our home, and treated my family to dinner at home to celebrate. He told me how proud he was of my accomplishments. It truly felt so good to have that support from my mate.

I also made a conscious decision to date in front of my Son-shines so they could see the process of choosing someone who is best for you instead of settling for the first person who shows interest in you. I explained to them dating didn't mean having sex. They were there to witness firsthand my process, and they noticed how happy I became when Joe and I dated—the happiest I had ever been with any man. Deon even confirmed this in his speech at our wedding reception, saying he had never seen his mother so happy, and Joe had taught him how to be a man.

I was always rushing and when Joe and I began our life together, he would constantly tell me to slow down. I was so used to running errands with my children, for my children, and anyone else I helped that I didn't walk or do much of anything at a moderate pace. Additionally, I aimed to be punctual by consistently practicing being on time for all events. A single parent with multiple children does not have the luxury of idle time, and multi-tasking became my norm. I was so used to this pace that I didn't even recognize I was doing it until Joe began telling me to slow down. I felt that if I didn't do everything for my children, who could I count on? Joe proved through his actions that he is reliable and capable. He lifted the weight off my shoulders and lightened my burden. I then was freed to take better care of myself and be a good woman to him.

Joe surprised me by proposing to me on December 22, 2018, in the basement of our home, surrounded by our children and our families. I felt an intense sense of emotion at that moment; although I cannot recall his exact words as he knelt before me, I do remember that he proposed marriage and expressed a lifelong commitment. I'm notoriously not emotional, so it was a big deal when I cried. I am so thankful that I never gave up on love or how I wanted to be loved. I thank God I worked on myself to be deserving of this love. I am thankful that our children can see us loving each other in our home in a healthy way, maybe not perfect but healthy.

We decided to get married at Markham Courthouse on August 23, 2019, in front of family and close friends. We both dressed casually for our courthouse wedding. I wore an off-white A-line dress, and he wore a buttoned-up shirt, blazer and jeans. Our children were all present except Jojo because it wasn't our court ordered time with him. Joe got us to a party bus that night, mostly for us and his out-of-town family from Missouri, including his father who I call Papa Joe. The party bus picked us up at our house and drove us to the city and around downtown Chicago, stopping at the Rock and Roll McDonalds and Buckingham Memorial Fountain to take pictures and dance. The next day, August 24, 2019, we had a beautiful wedding reception with over two hundred guests—all family and friends there to witness us jumping the broom. We swore to one another that we would never give up on each other, no matter what. We would fight together, not against each other.

Our children made up our wedding party, my brother Elijah was our emcee, and Aireale agreed to give us a toast and share her sentiments since I credited her for meeting him. Joe's cousin Anita also shared words to toast representing his side of the family. JaNiya and Deon shared beautiful expressions of love and unity representing our children. I asked other married couples in our families to open our reception with a couple's dance to whatever song they chose. It was as a testament to what Joe, and I were joining in holy matrimony like these couples. I'Esha and Vexton Buggs and Shantea and Ganell McCain ushered in the spirit of love as couples who have been together well over twenty years. We both have learned so much wisdom from watching them.

My cousin James and his beautiful wife Shira said the prayer before dinner. James has passed away since and I miss him every day. I miss talking, texting, and praying with him.

As a wife, I work on being the best I can to Joe daily. I pray for him and our children daily. My focal point is trusting God for our marriage. I love being challenged to become my highest self and I enjoy watching Joe get better as a husband. I learned to view my family as teammates, not opponents, and stopped trying to "win" arguments. By listening to understand and focusing on personal growth, I aim to have a positive impact on loved ones and build character and maturity as I seek wisdom.

In October of 2019, I received a lateral promotion at work from auditing to working a congressional position with the Department of Treasury in Joint committee. It was a welcome change for me to expand my knowledge in other areas of the tax code within the department of treasury.

In February 2020, my handsome brother Elijah wed the beautiful Samantha on a gorgeous rooftop in Phoenix, Arizona. I was asked to say some inspirational words, and I was obliged with Joe standing on my side. I quoted 1 Corinthians 13:4-7:

> Love is patient, love is kind. It does not envy, it does not boast, it is not proud. It does not dishonor others, it is not self-seeking, it is not easily angered, it keeps no record of wrongs. Love does not delight in evil but rejoices with the truth. It always protects, always trusts, always hopes, always perseveres.

They had a beautiful wedding and reception filled with love from family and friends.

In March 2020, COVID-19 shut the world down. We were now living in a pandemic. No sports, no traveling, no visitors, no one going anywhere. School was closed; offices were closed except for essential workers like those in healthcare, grocery stores, fast food, and emergency municipalities. I was already working from home mostly, so the mandate wasn't an issue for me.

During this time, Sugarplum would come over to visit after we both had been tested for COVID-19 and had a clean bill of health. We spent quality time cooking, eating, talking all night. She taught me how to take care of my plants and report them. We talked about our future and empowered one another with great laughs in between. I gleaned so much knowledge when we spent time together that our conversations always make me feel better and seen. I don't have to explain myself because she gets me. I don't have to apologize for my choice because she doesn't judge. I didn't have any issues of dimming my light around her because she never took my accomplishments like bragging or competition, which allowed me to shine even more. I attended both of her graduations from Northwestern University for undergrad and grad. She loved seeing me win because she had been there from the start. I had the same relationship with my dearly departed cousins, Karen and Dominique. The relationship Sugarplum and I shared was like big sister to little sister, and I valued it greatly. I couldn't wait for her to find her person, the love of her life, and see her blossom. She deserves all the love that she gives.

MAKING FAITH MOVES

A therapist told me once, "Cassandra, you will not die from a broken heart, so I want you to date without your boundaries and defense mechanisms." I chose to do that with a guy I dated

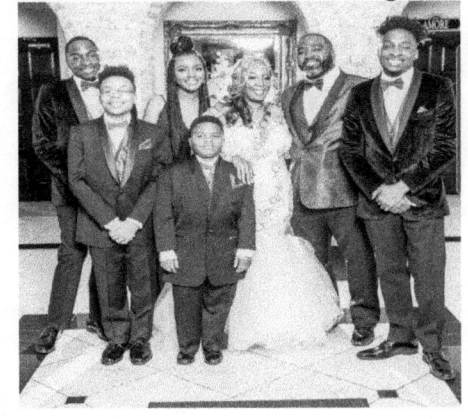

before I met Joe, and that relationship taught me so much that it helped me be a better woman and wife for Joe. I allowed my heart to open, trusted love without my usual safety net, and experienced heartbreak. That breakthrough assisted me tremendously when it came to love. I no longer believed in "hurting them before they hurt me." I now understood the power and privilege of love and being in love with a real man. It took faith and did work on myself. I had to grow up, gain emotional intelligence, and be willing to give grace.

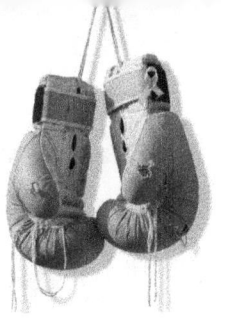

CHAPTER 14

Toni Morrison:
"YOU WANNA FLY, YOU GOT TO GIVE UP THE SH*T THAT WEIGHS YOU DOWN."

On April 12, 2021, I felt a lump in my right breast as I was drying off from a shower. I stepped into our bedroom and asked Joe to feel it. He said, "*You need to call your doctor.*" I did. When no one answered, I left a voice message. Two days later, I was telling my sister Maxine about the lump, and she said, "*You better call your doctor.*" I said I did, and no one answered. "*Call them again!*" I called and made an appointment to come in the following day.

They confirmed what I felt in my right breast and scheduled a biopsy for Wednesday. They said my doctor would contact me with the results by Monday. Instead, she called me Friday, April 23, 2021.

Hello, it's Breast Cancer...

On Friday, April 23, 2021, I was waiting in the car pick-up line at Zion's middle school and was chatting with my bond-sister Shantea. Our bond is not blood, but it is even stronger than that. Ten minutes into our conversation, my other line started beeping.

I clicked over to answer, and it was my doctor, Dr. Scott-Terry, who said she had the results.

"Hello, Cassandra, how are you today?"

"I am doing well Doctor, how are you?"

"Cassandra, I am calling to inform you of the results from your biopsy. you have Breast cancer. "

I took a deep breath. A single tear fell from my left eye, and my voice cracked as I asked:

"What stage?"

"Preliminary stage 3; however, we don't know for sure until other tests and maybe surgery."

"Do you recommend anyone or any hospital?"

"There are two Doctors I can recommend, one is close, and the other is further away."

"I would like to go to the best, regardless of how far away."

"One is at advocate where you went for the biopsy, and the other is located at the cancer treatment center in Zion, Illinois."

"I must let my husband know my test results before making my choice."

My doctor let me know she didn't usually give her patients her personal cell phone number, but she provided it and asked me to call her back after discussing with my husband so she could set it up. I assured her I will. I clicked over to Shantea and told her what my doctor told me. She was silent. I told her I had to call Joe; she understood and said, "I love you sister" as always. I was still ten minutes early to pick up Zion. Joe didn't answer my calls; he worked the night shift and was probably sleeping. I didn't want to leave a message. I needed to tell him this now, so I made a U-turn from the pick-up line headed back to wake Joe. My heart was in my stomach, and my stomach was in knots.

I pulled into the driveway, raised the garage door, pulled into the garage, turned the car off and went into the house headed straight to my bedroom where I left Joe sleeping.

He was sleeping so well; I didn't want to wake him. I gently shook his legs. I kissed him on the forehead. He opened his eyes with a start.

> "Baby, my doctor called me with my results of the biopsy. She said I have breast cancer, baby."

DEAD SILENCE.

Joe looked at me with sad disbelief in his eyes. I put my arms around his neck as he sat up, and we cried together. I assured him God already told me he had me, and we would be all right. I consciously breathed in and out to make sure I kept breathing. Joe got out of bed, and I said we had to pick up Zion. As he dressed, he was distraught, tears spilling from his eyes. I held his hand as we walked out our bedroom, down the hallway, past our children's bedrooms to the four stairs leading to the main level. We walked slowly through the living room and the dining area and the kitchen to the garage. I drove to Zion's school in silence, picked him up, explained why we were late, and drove us home as normally as possible. I stopped Zion before he went to his room to say I had the results of the biopsy. His eyes indicated he was afraid as he asked me what they were. It was positive for breast cancer. He hugged me with tears in his eyes.

> "Everything is going to be all right, Son-shine."

I told him we trust God especially for tough times like these. We embraced in the kitchen until we calmed down. When I released him from my hug, he went to his room, needing alone time. I allowed him to take time processing while Joe smoked a Cuban cigar and had a drink in the garage. I told him we had to call my doctor back together to discuss treatment options.

Together in the garage, we called the doctor back from my cell phone. She immediately expressed her prayers to us for this journey. Her sentiments were so warm and calming. We decided on the Cancer Treatment Center and called her associate and let us know they would be contacting us for a consultation appointment in two weeks.

Two weeks? That's so long to wait to find out if I will live or die. What kind of breast cancer do I have? What will happen to me? All my grandparents passed away from cancer. Life just got mad real! I can't die. I'm only forty-four years old! I'm not done raising my children! I don't even have grandchildren yet! Joe and I just found each other. I had done what I was supposed to do so that now I could do whatever I wanted.

You can have 99 problems, but once your health is threatened you only have one.

I wasn't ready to die!!!!

I thought about how devastating this diagnosis would be for my children, my parents, and everyone who loved me. I didn't want to be the reason that anyone was sad.

I told Joe we have to tell our children, our parents, our family and friends. It was surreal. I didn't have the words to speak, couldn't formulate the sentence "*I have breast cancer.*" So, I sent everyone a text filled with hope.

The rest of the day was a whirlwind. My sisters, Maxine, Shantea, Nicole, and Belinda, all came over despite my texting that I didn't want any company. These heifers don't listen! Then Joe's cousin Aja and husband Derrick came over with breast cancer support gifts for me. I had no idea where Joe was while we were sitting in the basement. My mind was so cloudy.

I began journaling days ago to document my feelings and emotions, as I normally do for 40 days when necessary. I had no clue this was on the horizon. I began each journal entry with "Dear God," then I proceeded to pour out my heart, prayers, tears, pain, joy.

My sisters planned a surprise prayer brunch at the beginning of my battle; Shantea paid a family friend to bring the twins home from where they lived in Iowa. There was so much food and so many people came to my home to cover me and my family in prayer. My friend RaMeka and her husband Darryl were there, and Darryl led us all in prayer as I began my journey through battling breast cancer.

Joe and I chose to get my treatment at the Cancer Treatment Center in Zion. My first appointment date after being diagnosed was May 4, 2021, on my Great Grandmother's birthday. The drive was over an hour, and I think it was the quietest Joe, and I have ever been. I just looked out the window in disbelief, hoping that when we got there, they would say it's a miracle, the cancer is gone. That did not happen.

DIAGNOSIS

Joe and I walked in the building, checked in at the registration desk, took our name tags, and went where they told us. As we waited in the lobby with our masks on, surrounded by other patients and their caregivers, I was looking around and wondered if I looked sick. It was all so surreal to me because I had been healthy all my life until now. They called my name; Joe and I followed a lady to the back. She said she was part of the registration team and would check insurance, birthdate, schedule, wristband, and meal cards for the cafeteria. After registration, I went to the clinic to meet my care team: oncologist, nurse practitioner, surgeon, and oncologist plastic surgeon.

My oncologist explained that I was diagnosed with preliminary stage 3, but technically it was stage 2B Triple Negative Breast Cancer. She made a diagram of what that meant and advised me strongly against looking it up on the internet because it would only scare me. She said they have an aggressive plan because it is an aggressive cancer. The American Cancer Society states, "Triple-negative breast cancer accounts for about 10-15% of all breast cancers. These cancers tend to be more common in women younger than age 40, who are Black, or who have a BRCA1 mutation."

Ai explains triple negative breast cancer (TNBC), also known as basal-like breast cancer, is a type of breast cancer that lacks estrogen and progesterone receptors and does not overproduce the HER2 protein. It's characterized by rapid growth, a higher risk of metastasis before diagnosis, and a tendency to recur compared to other breast cancers. TNBC accounts for about 10-15% of all breast cancer cases. TNBC is known for its faster growth rate and higher tendency to spread to other parts of the body compared to other breast cancer types. TNBC has a higher risk of recurrence compared to other breast cancer types, according to Mayo Clinic.

PROGNOSIS

They would need to perform another biopsy along with other tests to make a clear plan based on the data. Due to its unique characteristics, TNBC can be more challenging to treat than other breast cancers, as it does not respond well to hormone therapy or therapies targeting HER2. The oncologist informed me I would have to undergo 16 rounds of chemo and after the second treatment, I would lose all my hair. She told me the first four would be biweekly and twelve of the chemotherapy would be every week, but it was a milder form. She also told me of my options regarding surgery and removing the tumor: they can do a lumpectomy instead of removing my breast(s). I told her I wanted both removed. Was I sure, she asked, because the cancer had not spread beyond my breast. I was certain. She then explained I would need 25 rounds of radiation therapy to eliminate any remaining cancer cells to ensure the cancer did not come back. It would get hard and painful, she said, but they were here to make sure it was as painless as they could make it. When did I want to begin treatment? I said today.

My insurance cleared everything. I did another biopsy, which was painless unlike the first one. They inserted a marker next to the 1.6 cm breast tumor to find it more easily, and then I was told I had a 1-cm tumor under my arm. My diagnosis got very real. They would not only give me medicine, but I would have an apparatus INSIDE my body called a power port. A Power Port is a type of implantable port, a small medical device placed under the skin, typically in the chest area. It's designed to provide repeated access to the bloodstream for treatments like chemotherapy or IV infusions, and it's also MRI-compatible. Power Ports are often used by patients needing regular access to their vascular system, such as those undergoing chemotherapy or requiring long-term IV medication.

I couldn't wait until they were done with inserting my power port so I could run into Joe's arms, I was so sad for myself. The shock and numbness were wearing off. I was entering the stages of grief. I could feel Joe was too. There was so much said without words between us that day. The pain we both felt was loud. While waiting, I lay my head on his shoulder. As we walked between appointments, he held my hand. After my pre-op for my port placement, I had an appointment to speak with the chaplain. I almost fainted: Lord, am I going to die now? A chaplain makes reality almost too real. It hit me like bricks: I was fighting something that could easily kill me, and there was no coming back from that. The chaplain asked if I wanted an in-person visit or would telephone suffice? I thought to myself: You tell me, *can* this be over the phone? That would mean I wasn't about to die, because if I really was terminal, it would be in person. "*Telephone is fine*," I said, and he began praying for my healing.

I then headed to surgery to insert my port. As they prepped for me, a nurse walked me through the procedure. Before I went under anesthesia, she mentioned I had a good spirit and attitude. "*Keep mind over matter and you will be successful*," she said.

That was it. Mind over matter, and I would win. I made up my mind that was how I would fight this disease. I remembered the nurse who told me to hold on to my faith when I gave birth to my premature twins. I held on to my faith then, and I would do so again.

I had more appointments, and by the time we finished the first day, we were emotionally drained. We stayed at a hotel down the street from Center. Every step I took was heavy, the day dragged first but then passed quickly. Too much to process. The thoughts never stop.

Before we went to bed, I texted our support team of family and friends who were anxious to hear about my day. Day two was more of the same, with appointments to check my brain, my heart, my lungs, and my genes. They tested my genes and noticed I tested positive for RAD51. RAD51 expression has been linked to aggressive forms of triple-negative breast cancer and lymph node metastasis. Women with a RAD51C mutation have about a 10-15 percent lifetime risk for ovarian, fallopian tube or primary peritoneal cancer (these three cancers and their risks are related and are often referred to together as ovarian cancer). I informed my family, specifically the women in my bloodline of this cell mutation so they can get tested as well. This meant I would need to consider surgery to remove my ovaries as a cancer risk reducing procedure.

TREATMENT

Doxorubicin (AC chemo) is the first Chemotherapy included in my treatment plan, for four sessions, every two weeks. It is well known for difficult side effects in most cancer patients, especially nausea and vomiting, hair loss, low blood cell counts, and mouth sores. Doxorubicin is powerful, and the side effect are so intense, they are named for Satan himself, and not just because of their bright red color. It changes your urine red too for the first 24 hours. The drug is commonly called the "red devil chemo" because of its distinctive color and the evil effects it can create, including potential heart damage in some individuals. My oncologist carefully tested me to see if I was vulnerable to the heart effects. Doxorubicin is one of the most powerful chemotherapy options for a wide range of cancers. Because of the way it works, it can kill cancer cells at any point in their life cycle and stops cells from reproducing. When a cell unwinds its strands of DNA to replicate, doxorubicin attaches itself to the DNA, putting itself between the DNA and the enzyme needed for replication. The lower levels of platelets and red and white blood cells may lead to other side effects, such as looking pale and risk of bleeding.

The second form of chemotherapy that was included in my treatment plan was Taxol, also known as paclitaxel, I was to be given weekly for 12 rounds. Taxol is used to treat various cancers, including ovarian, breast, lung, esophageal, Kaposi's sarcoma, cervical, and pancreatic cancer. Taxol is a mitotic inhibitor, meaning it disrupts the process of cell division (mitosis), ultimately leading to cancer cell death. Specifically, it binds on microtubules, which are essential for cell division, and prevents them from functioning properly. This disrupts the separation of chromosomes during cell division, hindering cell growth and replication. Common side effects of Taxol include Hair loss: This is a common and temporary side effect. Bone marrow suppression: This can lead to a decrease in blood cell counts, increasing the risk of infection, anemia, and bleeding. Numbness and tingling: Also known as peripheral neuropathy, this can affect the hands and feet. Allergic reactions: Some individuals may experience allergic reactions. Muscle pains and diarrhea: These are also potential side effects.

Both radiation therapy and chemotherapy work by destroying cancer cells, but they do so in different ways. With chemotherapy, drugs target and kill cancer cells or stop them from dividing, while radiation therapy delivers high-energy X-rays to destroy cancer cells.

My first chemotherapy infusion was overwhelming. They checked my port, as they would do for each to make sure it was working. They checked all my vitals before setting me up in the room for chemo. I pulled out my adult coloring books which proved to be so relaxing and exactly what I needed in a hard season. The nurse explained all the meds they would administer to my port today, including meds to help with nausea, steroids to help with the pain, and AC chemo. The nurse had on a full hazmat suit with gloves to administer this medication. Let that sink in for a moment. They were giving me something so potent and harmful that the nurse could not touch it, but this potion would keep me alive. It would kill *all* my cells, both good and bad. I sat for 2.5 hours with Joe by my side, coloring, not thinking of my current circumstances but looking towards a future of healing. Mentally I couldn't stay there. It was too much. Too many thoughts. After my chemo infusion, Joe and I went home, mostly silent but listening to the music. I was waiting to feel something from my chemo.

SIDE EFFECTS

Some side effects I experienced included anemia, bleeding gums, mouth sores, fatigue and weakness, loss of appetite, hair loss, constipation, fever, changes in heart rate, weight loss, nail discoloration (with blackish dots on each nail!), stomach/abdominal pain, and dizziness.

A complication when receiving doxorubicin is leakage out of the vein into the surrounding tissue. This caused a blister on my buttocks, what I was told was extravasation. I was treated with elevating the site and setting a dry, cold compress on the site for 20 minutes, then applying honey on the wound. People can develop heart problems for a few months or up to 20 years after getting doxorubicin, so I began taking CoQ2 vitamins to help strengthen my heart.

The first day after receiving chemotherapy I had good energy, however by day 3 I was unbelievably exhausted it felt like I had been hit by a bus. I could barely walk from my bed to my bathroom. My body ached; it even hurts to drink or eat anything. I had no appetite. If I ate or drank, my body vibrated pain through my bones. My chest ached weirdly, so we went to the ER. They checked and I left. Little did I know I had a blood clot on my heart, which would soon be discovered by my care team. I would think about my great grandmother, Flora, that went through this, and my Grandma Janet. I gained strength from God and them to fight with all I had inside me.

Joe and I discussed whether I should take time off from work during the next four months of chemotherapy. I didn't want to, but when I listened to my body, I agreed with Joe. My manager, Celeste, was so supportive and started my paperwork, discussed the Family Medical Leave Act, and set me up to request and receive donated leave from my colleagues since I didn't have enough accumulated leave to take off with paid leave for four months. My colleagues donated 150 hours of leave to me anonymously, so I didn't miss any paycheck during my leave. I am eternally grateful for everyone that donated hours of their hard earned leave to me in my time of need.

I joined a breast cancer support group on Facebook that provided valuable support, information regarding symptoms, and a sense of community. I received encouragement and assistance from members through posts, comments, and private messages, many of which included prayers that I retained for reference. Additionally, thoughtful gifts were regularly sent to my home. Throughout my experience, I maintained resilience, focus, and clear boundaries, relying on guidance and discernment throughout the process.

After years of nonstop responsibilities since having twins at 22, I struggled to rest and let others care for me, feeling uneasy about needing help. We hired a cleaning team for our home because I could no longer do that. My body felt as if it weighed a ton and walking across the room was like walking a mile. Every move I made had a sigh or sound attached. I sounded like Michael Jackson oohing, ahhing, uhhing with every move. I took my meds as prescribed.

After reviewing relevant information, we chose to switch to a cleaner diet. I eliminated carbonated drinks, processed food, and sugar from my diet as much as possible, along with fried foods. I ate mostly fruit and vegetables and drank alkaline water. I drank green tea with honey, soursop tea with pineapples, fish and light meats. I lost thirty pounds in one week because I had no appetite, and it hurt my body when I tried to eat and drink anything. I felt aches in my back from my neck on down that would radiate and throb when I ate or drank. I went from 180 pounds to 150 pounds so quickly. I was also on a diet of only good energy, no extra stress or drama. For days, I sat quietly looking out my window at the sky, the trees, the sun and the moon allowing God to work.

After my first chemo, my hair began coming out when I combed it, by the second treatment it came out in patches so much that I had to contact my hair stylist and friend, Paulette, to come over and shave it off. As Zion's 8th grade graduation approached, I aimed to maintain a healthy appearance for his special day. Paulette, accompanied by her assistant, Mish, visited to review my hair situation. During the process, Paulette offered a prayer and displayed strong emotion as she shaved my hair. Mish observed quietly, managing her feelings with composure. I knew they were trying their best not to break down and cry in front of me. I remained collected and reassured them both that everything would be alright. Afterwards, Paulette spoke with me and expressed her admiration for my chosen approach to confronting this challenge. She noted that I had options and commended my decision to face the situation with a positive attitude. Paulette remarked on my resilience and presence, observing that I maintained a noticeable vitality despite the circumstances. Before departing, she offered support and prayed with me. I contacted a makeup artist, Wendy, that Paulette recommended to make my face for Zion's 8th grade graduation. She came over and made me look beautiful; I didn't want my son to be embarrassed on his big day.

Each waking day when I looked in the mirror, I couldn't recognize the person looking back. I didn't know who or what to expect from day to day. I lost all the hair on my head, eyebrows, eyelashes, my whole body. My mouth sores, burned tongue, black fingernails, my skin texture was rougher and my hue darkened. I lost toenails. I felt and looked ugly. I was so shocked that I snapped photos and told my sisters I looked like the character from *The Fly*. I joked that my ear might fall off just like his. On days I had energy, I listened to music and danced. When I couldn't leave my bed, I gave myself grace and stayed coloring, thankful for all my family and friends that sent me adult coloring books. During this period, I felt compelled to write as visions of my future emerged, which unsettled me. Observing nature each day helped me recover from exhaustion and pain, ultimately leading to unexpected growth.

On one occasion, the discomfort from chemotherapy was severe enough to interrupt my sleep. I sat on the edge of my bed until I felt steady enough to walk to the bathroom, taking care not to disturb Joe as he rested. To manage persistent back pain, I maintained a quiet routine during these episodes. I consistently kept my Yeti water bottle with me, and our family friend Rodney regularly delivered large quantities of Alkaline water to our home. I would quietly shut the bathroom door and sit on the toilet, praying and rocking, praying and drinking water.

One time when I showered, I had to call Joe to help me finish because I had no energy and thought I would pass out. Losing my independence was painful. I was used to being self-sufficient. The totality of this illness was so voluminous I had to break it down into pieces to dissect and execute a plan of keeping my sanity and holding on for dear life to my faith.

Some nights I couldn't sleep at all so I would sit in the front room, watching dawn turn into day.

During my second chemotherapy session, my father accompanied us. Due to significant physical weakness, I was unable to walk unsupported. Joe assisted me from the car and provided a wheelchair, after which my father transported me inside as we prepared for the day's appointments. The oncologist evaluated my blood laboratory results, vital signs, and port. An elevated heart rate, breathing difficulties, and chest pain were noted, prompting immediate transfer to the emergency room for further assessment. That was when they discovered the mass sitting on my heart. They treated it like a blood clot in the heart, also known as coronary thrombosis, which can block coronary arteries, leading to a heart attack (myocardial infarction).

The clot restricts blood flow, depriving the heart muscle of oxygen and potentially causing damage. Symptoms can include chest pain, shortness of breath, and discomfort in the upper body. Prompt treatment is crucial to prevent severe complications. I couldn't get my chemo infusion at this visit because I had an infection and needed to return in two weeks for more of the AC chemo "red devil." They treated the blood clot on my heart by prescribing me with blood thinners, often Joe had to administer it to me in the form of a shot.

After four rounds of the "red devil," I was treated with Taxol chemotherapy for nine weeks. Taxol interferes with cancer cell division. It uses solvents to dissolve paclitaxel, the main ingredient, so the medicine can enter the bloodstream. These solvents may make Taxol difficult to tolerate. Taxol chemo can lower white blood cells, which helps your body fight infections.

Having a lower blood cell count can make it easier for you to bleed from an injury. Like almost all breast cancer medicines, Taxol has miserable side effects. The low white blood cell counts left me susceptible to infection, so my care team placed the Neulasta medication on my belly with a scheduled time release to stimulate bone marrow to produce new blood cells. This process was painful, so I took steroids and rested. I also experienced neuropathy or numbness in my fingers and toes. Neuropathy, or nerve damage, in fingers and toes can manifest as peripheral neuropathy, which often affects extremities. Symptoms can include numbness, tingling, burning sensations, sharp pain, and muscle weakness. The neuropathy pains in my hands and feet became too unbearable to continue with the chemotherapy so I stopped after nine rounds of Taxol instead of twelve.

I completed my chemotherapy infusions on September 14, 2021, after a total of thirteen treatments instead of sixteen as originally planned. September 17th marks my cousin Karen's birthday, and I found the week of her birthday to be symbolically significant as it coincided with the completion of my chemotherapy treatment. My medical team, including physicians and nurses, showed support as I rang the bell alongside Joe, and they presented a certificate to mark my completion of chemotherapy. As emotional as I was, I still couldn't cry because I knew I had more work to do. Me and Joe shared a special moment that part one of this healing journey was behind us. I celebrated every win with my tribe. All my family and friends called or texted me to congratulate me on ringing that bell. My sisters: Maxine, Shantea, Nicole and Belinda and mother planned a surprise when we arrived at our house, they were waiting with little bells to ring the bell with me, with food, love and support. Zion conveyed his pride in my successful completion of chemotherapy. My twins called from their home in Iowa to celebrate this milestone with me and shared the concerns they experienced throughout my treatment, noting that offering prayers was all they could do. I assured them that this support was more than sufficient. JaNiya contacted me from Kentucky to extend her congratulations on completing chemotherapy. My Sugar Plum, Tinesha, Tee and Auntie Mimi called me emotionally over my completion of chemotherapy, they shared how proud they were of me. My father, Yvonne, Elijah and Sammy facetimed me all together ringing the bell.

Additionally, my siblings, aunts, cousins and countless friends communicated their excitement through calls and messages all that day. Friends Tekeia, Ketari, Angel, Sheronda, Esha, Toya, Sheree, Ta'Shara, RaMeka, Natasha, Chanita and Chakeesha prayed, visited and sent me thoughtful gifts in recognition of this accomplishment as they did throughout this battle. My friend, Jafrika offered to take me to chemo to help us out, but Joe respectfully declined noting that he will take care of his wife. So, instead she came to pick me up when I was sick so I could get some air.

During this process, I consistently experienced a strong sense of support and was never isolated. This level of encouragement is extremely valuable and cannot be overstated. We remain grateful to all who offered their presence and assistance during a period when I faced significant personal challenges.

Our oncologist urged us to take a break and even a trip after finishing chemotherapy before starting radiation. The weight of this illness stays with you in every thought, every ache, every minute. Joe and I chose to visit Playa Majeures in Mexico for a five-day/four-night, adults-only all-inclusive vacation in September 2021. I felt insecure, looking ill and worrying that Joe had to vacation with me in this state. I appeared more like a patient than his partner. Outwardly, I seemed confident and cheerful, but internally I struggled with intense emotions as my body changed, and my clothes no longer fit properly. Nothing flattered me, and I had to match my outfits with my bald head. I needed to rest enough to even walk and travel, but I was willing to build myself up just to see the sun and water on our vacation. I traveled with so much medication, including blood thinners for the clot on my heart. Nonetheless I was grateful to be alive, so I put on my smile and planned to enjoy my trip with my husband.

This excursion was my first trip abroad. Having a peaceful environment was important. I found solace standing in the water and feeling sand between my toes. I inhaled the fresh air and exhaled the pains in my body. I stretched my arms to the sun, thanking the Most High Father God for my life. I vowed to take better care of myself and stop trying to fix whatever I did not break.

At times, my actions may have led my loved ones to believe that I was indifferent or that my feelings were unimportant, as I frequently devoted my time, resources, and assistance to meeting their needs. I ignored my pain for so long that now it was time to correct my mistakes. That process would begin with acknowledging the abandonment of little Cassandra. As my body was transforming, so too was my mind.

In such vulnerable moments, I feel the presence of God the most. I lean on him when the pain is so great that I cannot even cry. I had to declare I had a life worth living just for myself. I was working myself into an early grave by trying to do God's job as if I was the Messiah. Instead, I had to do my job and let God do his. I was living like tomorrow was promised to me. Like I could help everyone else and then figure out how to help myself later. God tried to tell me back in 2011 when I had a TIA that I am not God and cannot save people. I could not continue giving 100% of myself to others without stopping to refuel in the healthy ways that mattered most.-

> Isaiah 43:2 NIV: When you pass through the waters, I will be with you; and when you pass through the rivers, they will not sweep over you. When you walk through the fire, you will not be burned; the flames will not set you ablaze.

A month after completing chemotherapy, I began radiation therapy, also called radiotherapy, which is another type of cancer treatment. This treatment uses beams of intense energy to kill cancer cells. Radiation therapy most often uses X-rays, but there are other types, including proton radiation. Modern methods of radiation are precise, beaming directly at the cancer while protecting healthy tissues from high doses of radiation. Radiation therapy can be given inside or outside of your body. The most common kind is external beam radiation therapy using a large machine called a linear accelerator. High-energy beams are aimed at a precise point on your body. Radiation therapy damages cells by destroying their genetic material which controls how cells grow and divide. Healthy cells may be damaged along with cancer cells during radiation therapy, but healthy cells can repair themselves more easily than cancer cells.

The goal of radiation therapy is to treat cancer while harming as few healthy cells as possible. After surgery, to stop the growth of any remaining cancer cells, adjuvant therapy is given. As you lie still, the linear accelerator moves around you, delivering radiation from several angles. The machine is adjusted just for you by your care team, delivering the precise dose of radiation to the exact point needed on your body. You do not feel the radiation as it is beaming, much like not feeling an X-ray. External beam radiation is an outpatient treatment, which means no need to stay in the hospital. Treatment is given five days a week over several weeks. It spreads out this way, so healthy cells have time to recover between sessions.

Sometimes only one treatment is needed to relieve pain or other symptoms from more advanced cancers. Each session lasted about 10 to 30 minutes, most of which was spent molding your body into the right position. During treatment, you lie on the table as you did during planning. After each radiation treatment, I would rub endless Aquaphor cream on my breast and surrounding areas. I worked at home during my five weeks of radiation and was treated on my lunch break.

I tested positive for COVID-19 while going to radiation, so my nurses said I could still come for my treatment if I felt up to it. I said, "I do. I'll see you tomorrow." They changed my time from early in the day to being the last patient coming via a different entrance. After I completed all 25 radiation treatments, I noticed a burn on my back where the treatments were done but, in front, it looked as if the radiation had burned right through me to the other side. Two weeks later, I felt the pain of severe burns. The skin in the treated area might become red, dry, itchy, or even blister, resembling a sunburn. My skin peeled; I could pull it off like rubber under my breast. I took pictures and kept rubbing cream to help.

After the radiation treatments were completed, it was time to remove the blood clot from my heart. The Center referred me to a surgeon at the University of Chicago Hospital who could grab the clot off my heart without cutting through my chest cavity. This was known as intracardiac thrombosis, removing a clot from an artery or vein. I made an appointment for consultation two weeks after radiation and informed the surgeon of my double mastectomy and completion of chemotherapy and radiation therapy. He said I was a tough cookie to endure all those treatments, especially 25 rounds of radiation. I told him simply, as I told Joe, "*I want this behind me. The sooner, the better.*"-

During a mechanical thrombectomy, a surgeon introduces special devices through catheters that can either macerate or suction out clots from within the blood vessel. The surgeon explained they would enter my body at three points: the right side of my neck, the right side of my breast, and the groin—all to grab the clot off my heart. He warned me I would be in extreme pain—a level of 10—when I wake from surgery, but they would try to reduce it to 5. I was physically present, but I did what I usually do when I got anxious: in my mind, I fast forward, past the climactic moment, through the pain, through to the end of the storm. That is where I have always found the sun to shine brilliantly. I allow my mind to rest there until pain has stopped.

MAKING FAITH MOVES

I had to rescue the little girl inside. I had to affirm her, apologize to her for not standing up for her when she was molested. I had reached the sad stage of trauma where I knew what happened had a tremendous cost, not only physically but mentally and emotionally. I had to reconcile the feelings I felt by protecting those that harmed me instead of recognizing the great pain they caused me. I sat exhausted at home listening to Greg O Quin's song, "That's What I Told the Storm." This song ministered to my spirit. The words empowered me to keep fighting. I had to let go of the issues and people weighing me down from ascending to my higher self. There's a saying to whom much is given much is required, however, it is often misinterpreted. I had not yet achieved where I was making enough to give, I was giving sometimes despite myself and my children. I was giving of myself and my financial resources as I struggled to get it for myself instead of from my overflow. I had not yet had an overflow to give yet I gave. I had to stop trying to make everyone's life as prosperous as I was making mine. I have also learned that people don't want what you give them, they want what you have. I earned my lifestyle paid in blood, sweat and tears.

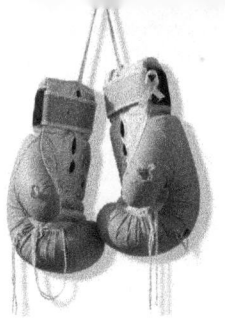

CHAPTER 15

Nas:
"TURNIN' NOTHIN' INTO SOMETHIN' IS GOD WORK, AND YOU GET NOTHIN' WITHOUT STRUGGLE AND HARD WORK."

"You don't get strong by standing at the finish line, you get strong with every step it takes to get you there." Toni Sorenson.

PTSD after cancer is more common than many people realize—and it's not just about the trauma of diagnosis. The entire cancer journey, from treatment to survivorship, can leave deep emotional scars.

What Is Cancer-Related PTSD?

Post-traumatic stress disorder (PTSD) can develop when someone experiences or witnesses a life-threatening event—like cancer. While many patients experience post-traumatic stress (PTS) symptoms, a smaller percentage develop full-blown PTSD. According to the National Cancer Institute, 3-4% of newly diagnosed patients and up to 35% of survivors show signs of PTSD.

Common Triggers and Symptoms

Cancer-related PTSD can be triggered at any stage:

- Diagnosis shock
- Intensive treatments or hospital stays
- Waiting for test results ("scanxiety")
- Recurrence fears
- Physical changes or side effects
- Symptoms may include:
- Intrusive memories or nightmares
- Hypervigilance and exaggerated startle response
- Avoidance of reminders (like hospitals or medical terms)
- Sleep disturbances and concentration issues
- Feelings of detachment or loss of interest in life

Treatment & Support Options

There are effective therapies:

Cognitive Behavioral Therapy (CBT): Helps reframe distressing thoughts and manage triggers

Eye Movement Desensitization and Reprocessing (EMDR): Targets traumatic memories through guided eye movements

Support groups: Offer connection and shared understanding

Mindfulness and relaxation techniques: Reduce anxiety and improve emotional regulation

Cancer survivors often feel pressure to "move on" or "be grateful," but emotional healing takes time. PTSD isn't a weakness—it's a valid response to a life-altering experience. If you or someone you know is struggling, reaching out to a mental health professional can be a powerful first step.

I had days when I confronted my mortality. Those were shattering. I had to admit I had an illness that had been terminal for so many of my loved ones: my great-grandmother, all my grandparents, Uncle Jobe. An illness that could take me away from my husband, my children, my parents, my life that I worked so hard to create. I understood the implications, but I refused to let it beat me. I had moments with God asking me if I wanted to live, not just for my children, my husband, my parents, my friends. But to live for myself. The ultimate fight was for my life, physically, spiritually, and mentally. I struggled with, "thy will be done", not sure if it was indeed God's will for me to fight this or not.

I updated our family after every appointment with a text. I just didn't feel like talking most days, I still struggle with this. I didn't keep my phone near me during this time, and people didn't like it if I didn't respond immediately to a call or text. My mind was all over the place. I was trying to find balance, hear answers from God on my direction and purpose. That requires stillness. I had to be still and listen. People would even get upset with Joe if he didn't respond. Joe had a lot to contend with at this time. I vented my frustrations to a chosen few: my Sugarplum, Aireale, my cousin Tinesha (whom I called (Petunia). They got livid and empowered me to ignore such selfish people. They reminded me I was fighting for my life and didn't owe anyone an explanation.

The support of family and the strength within were almost unreal. My husband took me to every chemo and doctor visit, took notes and asked questions that my mind was too cloudy to process often. My sister friend, Nicole, came over almost weekly to check on me. My Sugarplum, Auntie Mimi, and Big Sis Tanya were cautious of visiting due to COVID-19 and rightly so, but they brought masks, telephoned, texted, sent gifts, cried, laughed, or did whatever the day called for. My Aunt Mimi called and texted me often, sometimes breaking down each time I spoke with her. My Aunt Sharon, Aunt Jackie, and my uncles sent their love. My brother Elijah, his wife Sammy, his mother Yvonne, and my stepsister Ebony, all visited me from out of town. They were simply there, and it really meant a lot.

Joe's father, who I call Poppa Joe, and the Missouri family kept in communication, came to cook, and brought us a financial blessing. Poppa Joe came down from Missouri along with the Missouri family, Cousin Stevie and his wife Shondra, Cousin DaJuan and his wife Odessa, Cousin Paula, Auntie Renee, Cousin Sandreka, Zaya and Jay all visited, cooked, checked on us, and gifted us with blessings. Faithful cousins were ever present: Tee, Tinesha, Terry, Alex, Jobe, and Hollis. My brother Alonzo came over often to hang with Joe, and I appreciated everyone who helped distract him from the hard work of being my caregiver. My parents, my stepmother, my brother, and his wife visited and stayed with us to help us out. My Auntie Bettye visited frequently just to sit and talk with me even though she had health problems. She indulged me in great energy and hugs. My work mother, Inez, cooked us a feast for Thanksgiving with a caramel cake. My friends from work, Tawanda, Inez, and Mimi, visited with gifts. My Auntie Sharon, cousin/Sissy Tinesha, cousin Cake, sister, stepsister, cousin/brother Terry, Alex, Jobe, James, cousins Charles, Steve, Hollis, Nicole, Trina, Jermaine, Shaquila, and Toya frequently called or texted to check on me.

I noticed some people I thought would rally for me did not. It broke my heart to see that reality since I had sacrificed for people who could not do so for me. I worried about my Son-shines and their living conditions while living in Iowa. They struggled as young adults living on their own for the first time. I didn't want to prevent them from struggling because it builds character, I just wanted to help them manage their resources better. I worried more when they were home and hanging with people who were moving in the wrong direction. For the sake of my health, I couldn't concentrate on the negative, positive energy helps you heal faster. Instead, I chose to focus on all the people whose lives I've touched over the years who stepped up for me. I received cards, gifts, and meals, but especially prayers from friends spanning grammar school all the way up to my career colleagues. I was filled with gratitude for this showering of love. I prayed more and said less.

My parents were there for me the whole way, feeling my pain and sending support for me and Joe. They felt my pains and gave me and Joe so much support, I'm forever grateful God saw fit to allow my parents to be healthy during my health crisis.

However big or small the gesture is, I was thankful for all, even holding a gratitude brunch at my house on the anniversary of the day I was diagnosed April 23, 2023. I had Chef Maria on the menu and distributed thank you cards and breast cancer awareness ribbons to each guest.

In April, I had one of my two biannual oncology appointments to make sure I am still NED (No evidence of disease). I received great news on my body scans and saw wonderful numbers in my blood labs. I was filled with joy about my health outcome and all the people who had poured light into my darkest hours. I struggled to go from giver to receiver, but I learned how important it was to do so.

I prayed for Joe daily and told his friends not to worry about me but to take care of him. I knew what God told me, so I was living once again on my faith. The way Joe held me in bed at night, I knew he was afraid. He prayed for me, over me, confessing his undying love for me. I was glad the twins were not home at this time so they wouldn't have to see their superhero mom so down. They both visited home during this time and Deon even came back for a short while, and Joe helped him find a job. JoJo and JaNiya saw my experience in between their school obligations, but poor Zion saw it every day, especially at a time when he needed me so much. He was about to enter high school, meet lifelong friends, grow into a fine young man—these thoughts buoyed me as I fought to stay afloat. I was missing out on the crucial parts of my children's lives now, as if I had gone on pause while life kept playing around me. It felt unfair.

Throughout my treatment, I continued to fulfill my responsibilities as a parent. For instance, I communicated with JaNiya's high school counselors to ensure her inclusion in the National Honor Society, recognizing her dedication and the potential financial benefits for college. When Zion graduated from eighth grade shortly after my diagnosis, despite experiencing hair loss, I arranged for a company to deliver front-yard decorations that conveyed "Congratulations, Zion!" using his preferred colors. There were occasions when certain activities were not feasible; for example, I was unable to celebrate Zion's graduation in the same manner as I had with my twins or assist him with back-to-school shopping and registration. Nevertheless, I remained confident that there would be future opportunities to participate more fully. I had complete faith in that. I trust God will always bring me through; I have crazy faith!

MAKING FAITH MOVES

What has always meant more to me than dressing nicely is being a good person, with integrity and authenticity. Clearly, I understood this because every person I called a friend showed up for me throughout my breast cancer journey. To have good friends, you must first be a good friend in their presence as well as behind their back. They do not dim their light nor kiss my butt, they are not my fans, they have been my cherished friends, some of them, since elementary school.

I taught my children that what someone thinks of them is none of their business and certainly not their concern. Do not let criticism influence your emotions or attitude. Always consider the source of the information and decide if it is worth the concern. I factor in the various challenges individuals may face in their lives as well as their intelligence. With this understanding, I can often comprehend the reasons behind someone's decision to misrepresent or speak harshly about me. Sometimes when a person is not self-happy, they can deflect onto someone else in unkind ways. But life is filled with too many tests to waste time on anything or anyone who won't ever matter. Sometimes the favor in your life makes you shine so much it irritates those who choose darkness, don't let that bother you. Carry on and shine brightly like a diamond you're doing good work!

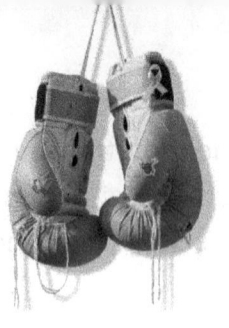

CHAPTER 16

Kendrick Lamar:
"SO NEXT TIME YOU FEEL LIKE YOUR WORLD IS ABOUT TO END, I HOPE YOU STUDIED BECAUSE HE'S TESTING YOUR FAITH AGAIN."

One day my chemotherapy pain woke me and got me out of my bed. I was in so much pain, I had to move around, so I walked over to the bathroom in our master bedroom quietly not to awaken Joe. I was weak and had lost thirty pounds. My breathing was labored. I sat on the toilet seat and leaned against the sink, feeling like I was no longer running but fighting I knew it was time to face my challenges head-on. I went from running a relay race to boxing. I felt I was in Round 12 of a vicious boxing match.

During a boxing match, a boxer encounters considerable physical stress due to repeated impacts, sustained exertion, and swift movements. Common physiological responses include muscular fatigue, increased heart rate, accelerated respiration, and occasional pain or discomfort resulting from strikes delivered by the opponent. Adrenaline can temporarily suppress the sensation of pain, which may enable individuals to continue activity despite injuries or fatigue.

At the same time, they must maintain intense concentration and strategic thinking under pressure. Anxiety, excitement, and the instinct to survive can cycle rapidly, leading to moments of high focus or emotional overwhelm.

Battling cancer felt like I was fighting a boxing match for my life. I feel like we must confront death and decide if you want to fight it, I chose to look the fear of death in the face and fight. I heard God telling me to fight. I believe I was experiencing what psychology today calls a near-death experience—the conscious, semi-conscious, or recollected experience of someone who is approaching or has temporarily begun the process of dying—such as during a cardiac arrest followed by resuscitation. People who recall near-death experiences have described perceiving a variety of surreal phenomena, like seeing themselves from above or passing through a tunnel of light. I can't recall everything that happened at that one moment, but I know I heard my Grandma Janet's voice: She used to tell us that if we were fighting someone bigger than us, we had to pick up something to knock them out. In that moment in my bathroom, I had to heed her words. I had to pick up something to fight for my life. God was indeed working for my greater good, but I had to put in work too. I had been allowing God to carry me through my battle, but now he was saying I had to fight. I had to don the full armor of God and gather my sword of faith. It felt like I had a large bat and swung it directly at the devil's head to get it away from me and knock him out. I was indeed fighting for my life.

Ephesians 6:10-18, NIV, explains the armor of God:

Finally, be strong in the Lord and in his mighty power. Put on the full armor of God, so that you can take your stand against the devil's schemes. For our struggle is not against flesh and blood, but against the rulers, against the authorities, against the powers of this dark world and against the spiritual forces of evil in the heavenly realms. Therefore, put on the full armor of God, so that when the day of evil comes, you may be able to stand your ground, and after you have done everything, to stand. Stand firm then, with the belt of truth buckled around your waist, with the breastplate of righteousness in place, and with your feet fitted with the readiness that comes from the gospel of peace. In addition to all this, take up the shield of faith, with which you can extinguish all the flaming arrows of the evil one. Take the helmet of salvation and the sword of the Spirit, which is the word of God.

Let me tell you, once you face the ultimate fear; fear of death, NOTHING else scares you. Even though the anxiety comes often, I fear nothing. I trust that everything will work out according to the will of God for my life and those connected to me. I live in the day to day, not stressing about tomorrow.

So, once again…Faith without works is dead. I could have just kept leaning on God through the pain. But instead, I heard him ask me to join him in a battle. It was up to me to claim ownership in the fight for my life. I had to start to speak up and show up!

My father called me about two days later. He said he felt my pain. He had become so overwhelmed with emotions at the same time I was experiencing this agony. We both cried tears of joy on the phone because I had made it through the near-death experience I shared with him.

I confronted mortality and embraced my vulnerability after I was done with all my treatments. As I fought my battle with cancer, I felt as if God had me in a coma. WebMD describes a coma as "a prolonged state of unconsciousness. During a coma, a person is unresponsive to their environment. The person is alive and looks like they are sleeping. However, unlike in a deep sleep, the person cannot be awakened by any stimulation, including pain. I was oblivious to anything around me and even within me. I didn't feel the weight of my breast cancer battle until I completed all my treatments. I endured 13 rounds of aggressive chemotherapy, a double mastectomy, 25 rounds of radiation, surgery to remove the blood clot from my heart, 11 hours of reconstructive surgery Part 1 (Diep flap), four hours of reconstructive surgery Part 2. I had four surgeries within a two-year period. That is a lot for the body to endure and recover from, and not once did I break down and cry. The pain was so severe, I couldn't cry.

One day as Joe and I were lying in bed watching a movie, I began scrolling Instagram on a commercial. We saw a couple on a TV series called Black Love. The wife had passed away from brain cancer. We watched the video her husband put together, and that was when I broke down. I cried, I cried loud. I was overcome with emotions. Tears flowed; my body rocked. It felt like I was finally waking up from my coma and now the reality of what I just endured hit me. I had been holding in so much pain. Joe rubbed my back as I cried, and he encouraged me to let it out. It took some time to allow the depths of my pain to appear in the form of tears instead of keeping it all in and internally hurting. I let all my anxieties, my worries, my stress, my fears and my victories out all at once that day and it felt so good. It was a cleansing that I indeed needed.

It felt as if I was crying for the little girl inside me that I had buried after she was molested; for the teenager and young woman inside me who had been raped twice and silent about it; for the single mother inside me raising three sons who struggled; for the survivor inside me who faced breast cancer. I wept because I never stood up for myself. I wept because I felt guilty for allowing myself to endure so much pain silently. I released all my emotions. It was liberating to let this part of myself out, finally and completely. I cried until my body stopped rocking and Joe held me, giving me a soft place to land. I felt free. I could inhale and exhale. I couldn't love Joe more at that moment. I was grateful. I am grateful that I have a man that can be tough, protects me and sensitive to my needs at the same time.

I began crying almost daily, not necessarily tears of sadness but tears of gratitude. I no longer thought of crying as a weakness, but as a strength and a cleansing. It takes strength to acknowledge you need help and ask for it. I was grateful to be here after a hard-fought battle. Once again, I knew God had saved my life again and I don't have plans on wasting this chance. Anything and everything God ask me or places before me will have a solid response: YES! However uncomfortable I get; I will pursue my God-given purpose until my last breath. I wrote out my personal mission statement with intentions and made a vision board.

Physical beauty is often linked to features like symmetrical faces, healthy skin, strong hair, and confident posture. For cancer survivors, these traits may be affected. After breast cancer treatment, I struggled with changes in my appearance. When I looked in the mirror, I only saw flaws, not beauty. I didn't like how my skin, my hair, my body had changed, so I worked hard on fixing me. I went to the dermatologist, and facials became a ritual to make my skin and face better. I constantly found products to help my hair. It was too dark, and my hair had thinned in the middle of my head. My hair stylist and friend helped color and strengthen it. Joe updated our gym membership, and I began going weekly until I went daily. I felt as if I was going through depression. I also realized that I had been functioning depressed when I was raising my sons as a single mother before I met Joe. As a result of experiencing depression and previous traumas, I found it difficult to recognize my own value or strengths. I relied on external validation for affirmation of my attributes. I once encountered an observation that butterflies are unable to see their wings and, consequently, cannot appreciate their own beauty; this analogy resonated with me, as I struggled to perceive my own positive qualities and questioned their existence. Recognizing this, I understood there was personal growth required. It is both an irony and a deep truth that those meant to encourage and inspire people are the ones who often struggle with self-esteem and issues with appearance.

Each day, my goal was to get up and shower, brush my teeth, wash my face, and look decent. I dressed up for all my doctors' appointments, chemotherapy, radiation, surgeries—even though this was a living hell, I didn't have to look like it.

One of the questions I asked my oncologist was if Joe and I could still have sex through my treatments and she affirmed that we could but would have to wait 24 hours after chemotherapy infusions.

I consciously tried to be present with all my children, giving them hope and wisdom through my battle. I made sure to pray for them individually because I knew they were hurting. They too did not want to burden me with their pain at seeing me fight cancer. Instead of showing them strength, I showed them transparency. No more masks that hide my emotions from them.

MAKING FAITH MOVES

I gained so much clarity during my time alone fighting this breast cancer battle. Every obstacle I encountered was a test of my faith. I prayed to pass the test so I wouldn't have to repeat the lesson. I knew I had been running fast and working hard ever since I gave birth to my twins. I thought about all the people I have helped and rescued by allowing them to live with me free of charge, paying their rent, minding their children, arranging their birthday parties, giving back to my community by volunteering my accounting services. I gave my mother all her milestone birthday parties since her 50th birthday and retirement party. I gave my children birthday parties according to their choice up until their 18th birthday. I worked hard every day fighting systemic racism in all areas of my life. I have given of my resources, talents, and time to assist others in any way I could. I donated money even when I didn't have it for my children. I made sure to save money for my children if I passed away in multiple life insurance policies. I did all of this while mostly being a single mother for years. I was more concerned with others' opinions than my own perspective. I tended to interpret things seriously and often responded defensively. I kept secrets of traumatic details done to me. I held in my feelings to not upset my loved ones. To avoid causing distress to others, I chose to internalize my feelings instead. Everything had to change, including me.

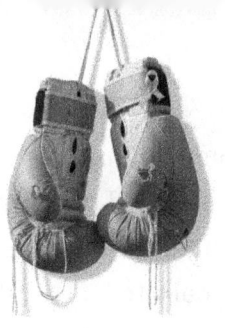

CHAPTER 17

Zora Neale Hurston:
"IF YOU ARE SILENT ABOUT YOUR PAIN, THEY'LL KILL YOU AND SAY YOU ENJOYED IT."

As I mentioned, after completing chemotherapy, Joe and I took a trip to Playa Mujeres, Mexico, so I could see the sun and water. When Joe and I were traveling back home from Mexico, we stopped to eat at the airport while waiting to board our flight. One reason we like to be early for our flights is to relax at the airport. We were sitting on stools at a restaurant when a young attractive couple sat next to us and began engaging us in small talk. They shared how they were heading home from a trip and how rejuvenated they felt from their vacation. They asked about us, and we shared our vacation details and how much we needed it.

The couple then showed off their matching tattoos, which read "Jeremiah 29:11," and explained what that scripture meant for them. I instantly got chills when I saw the tattoo. I had been silently praying to God to feel better about myself and asked for confirmation of some events. I shared with the couple that I used that scripture going through my recent battle with breast cancer. They commended me on my successful outcome and praised my efforts for overcoming the challenge. This felt like God confirming to me that I matter. I was seen instead of being overlooked as weak and insignificant. I feel I have matured spiritually to feel the discernment and messages God sends me daily. Everything happens for a reason. My heart is open to hear from God to guide and order my steps. Once you find that quiet and eliminate distractions, events get clearer. God showed me my purpose, and I vowed to pursue it until my last day on Earth. I choose to speak up for those in treatment, for those caregivers, for those hurting in any way, I choose to use my voice and speak up as loudly and as often as I can for those wounded in the areas I was. I am an advocate for all survivors with love, inspiration and on purpose.

My family had a first-class seat to witness my obedience to God. I was able to walk it like I talk it about faith in God. They all witnessed firsthand how prayer changes places and situations. They saw me fight for my life. They witnessed me in survival mode. Now they can see a softer version of myself. They saw me change my diet and my attitude because of this battle. I listen better now. I can apologize for my shortcomings and make amendments to do better instead of giving excuses for past behavior.

I carried the guilt of not choosing a good father for my Son-shines like the father I had. My father is a good dad present throughout my entire life, and, unfortunately, my Son-shines cannot say the same. For that reason, I have worked extra hard to provide for them. I had always been the caretaker for my children, but now I needed someone to care for me. I realized I had sheltered my boys, and now I knew that a leader must prepare their followers to lead. I had to teach them how to live without me, how to be self-sufficient.

That is so difficult. I had to step back and allow my twins to become the men I raised. Through their struggles, I trusted God for their lives and stepped back. I prayed so much and so hard for my children while redefining motherhood of adults in the face of adversity.

As I reflect on my entire life journey, I am grateful and in awe of how God has been turning it all around for me from the beginning. Yes, I experienced a lot of pain and heartbreak. However, once I began to trust God and stopped trying to fix everything myself, I discovered peace on an entirely new level. I had to mature, I had to heal, I had to forgive, I had to relearn, I had to readjust and realign my life to God and allow him total control. From my birth, childhood, and beyond, God has been faithful. I had no business thinking that I could go away to HBCU in Louisiana where I had no family and no money and still succeed! I took care of about 10 people in my twenties without charging anyone or taking advantage of them. I had no business thinking I could give birth and raise premature babies born at 26 weeks and finish college as an accounting major, but I did so! I had no business thinking I would survive Triple Negative Breast Cancer with a blood clot on my heart and still maintain my career and family! I had the audacity because I had faith in God and did the work to cultivate the life I wanted to live. God has been the constant in my life and kept me even when I had given up on myself. I allowed myself to be mistreated so badly that I lost myself. I thank God every day for his saving grace.

MAKING FAITH MOVES

I am healing out loud because I nearly died in silence. Each morning, I wake up with appreciation for the opportunity to start a new day. I begin by expressing gratitude for life, good health, my spouse, our children, parents, siblings, families, friends, home, transportation, love, peace, and safety. Practicing gratitude for one's circumstances is often considered an important foundation for a fulfilling life. The strength that God revealed I had in me is astounding—I still weep at the thought of it. Throughout my life, various factors have come together to provide support during challenging times. Barriers and distractions were removed, allowing me to focus on overcoming obstacles. My husband Joe was by my side to assist, and my parents remained healthy and able to offer help. I earned my MBA and took a lateral promotion to another division, which reduced my job stress.

Additionally, my children's needs were met, and we were able to purchase a comfortable home. I worried for my twins when they were young, especially given the risks young Black men face. They wanted independence, and I prayed they'd find a quieter place to grow into the men we raised them to be. I knew challenges would come, but that builds character, even if it's hard to watch sometimes. They will always be my babies. As a mother, I feel like my job is to nurture them forever, which looks like coddling! So, I have prayed often for God to protect my children. Send angels to surround them and let them know my love and support will always be available for them.

Throughout my life, I have consistently advocated for bodily autonomy and personal safety. As a Black American, I have also worked to secure fundamental rights such as life, liberty, and the pursuit of happiness. My efforts are not solely personal; they are intended to benefit all members of my community. Echoing Dr. Aireale's foreword and her reference to Fannie Lou Hamer, there is a collective sense of fatigue from longstanding injustices. Fannie Lou Hamer powerfully asserted, "Nobody is free until everybody is free." This principle continues to inspire and guide my commitment to equality.

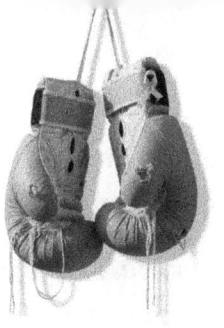

CHAPTER 18

Oliver Wendell Holmes: "WHAT LIES BEHIND US AND WHAT LIES BEFORE US ARE TINY MATTERS COMPARED TO WHAT LIES WITHIN US."

2 Thessalonians 3:3 NIV: But the Lord is faithful, and he will strengthen you and protect you from the evil one.

As I completed all my treatments, I found myself rushing to return to myself. I would explain why I looked how I looked to whoever I was around, wherever I went. I voluntarily shared my experience with breast cancer to total strangers. I know I still looked sick, bald, thin, weak. I walked slower because of lingering back pains from chemo. In fact, I became overly sensitive about how I looked. I knew I was trying to recover from trauma, so I contacted my therapist, Mrs. Janet, because I was overwhelmed mentally. Part of me needed to show I was in control showing exceptional progress, recovery—be the spokesperson for Best Breast Cancer Survivor. I don't like to fail at anything, and this was yet another opportunity to be "good at it." Can you imagine? I still did not let myself of the hook just to rest, relax, flow, let others give the care for a change.

Part of letting go is to resolve. I have resolved with anyone and everyone who has ever harmed me. I forgive them all, even those who never apologized for their cruelty. You must understand that there are people that are content with staying the same. Once they deem you think you are better than them, they will try to wage an attack against you and if they have no current access to your life, they will bring up your mistakes from your past to try to bring you back down to their level. They have no desire to grow so they won't learn their lessons nor recognize their mistakes. These people never acknowledge their faults and don't admit when they are wrong. They will team up with other people that see you as their competition to sabotage your character. Shade coming from a tree bearing no fruit should not bother you. I don't argue anymore, I adjust access to me and set boundaries to protect myself. My peace is more important than proving my point. You will never receive an apology but forgive them anyway. I don't offer this example to act like the bigger person. I do this because I have learned the hard way that I see them for who they are and not what I want them to be, which made it so hard for me to be around them.

I asked a family member to take my son (who graduated from 8th grade) and their graduate out to eat while I was sick and going through chemo treatments, offered to pay for the gas and the meal, they agreed to help but when the day came, they didn't do it. It hurt my feelings. Maya Angelou said, when people show you who they are believe them the first time. I have learned how my God works, sometimes he shows you repeatedly a person's heart towards you when you don't believe the first time. He had to break my heart to correct my vision, to prove to me they do not have good intentions concerning me. A wise man, Earl DMX Simmons, said see people as they are, trust them to be themselves. Expect a liar to be a liar, expect selfish people to be just that. Then place them accordingly.

I had a family member lie on me, and I instantly knew it was to tear down my integrity and sabotage my character because they did not like how other people showed me love so they wanted to dimmish that. There are people who don't like you because of the favor on your life. I no longer explain to those that should know me better what I would and wouldn't do. Before God elevates you, he's going to show you everyone's heart around you so you will know who to take with you and who to love from a distance. For my life, this means I do not include toxic people in my immediate circle, but I do place them where I can see them—keep my eye on them from afar. They are no longer in my front row of VIPs. My VIP section is for the ones who pray for me, love me in my authenticity, regardless of what I do for them. They are the ones who root for my future instead of reminding me of my past. They are positive people who care and feel concern without being told. They are servant leaders. They are who I aim to be and reciprocate—my own role models.

Each one of us is on our own individual assignment from God, which can be in every possible direction or, perhaps, just one definite path. No one matures at the same time in the same way for the same reasons. Therefore, I have multiple groups of friends—older, younger, married, single, some even far more mature than I. I learn something from each of them. I trust them to check me when I'm being reckless, and I promise not to get angry at the truth. I trust them not to compete with me but walk alongside me. I trust them with my reputation, my children, my family, my life. I expect this because I am doing this to all my family and friends. No doubt, I have done harm to others in my lifetime, but it isn't my core intention.

Separate a good person making a bad mistake from a bad person appearing good. I acknowledge my mistakes because each one has provided valuable lessons. Every less-than-shining moment was probably a source of learning that you won't ever forget or repeat. If you don't learn the lesson, you will surely repeat the test. Don't be angry about that, and don't stay angry about anything. Anger only harms. It is a choice as much as joy and peace are choices. Why not choose peace and joy?

> Hebrews 10:23 NIV: Let us hold unswervingly to the hope we profess, for he who promised is faithful.

I am still adjusting to my "new normal" after treatment, and I am hopeful. As I write this, I am a four-year cancer survivor and thriver. Each day I take a variety of vitamins and supplements to move my body and recharge my mind: turmeric, ginger, vitamin D3, vitamin B12, magnesium, lion's mane, oil of oregano, multivitamin, elderberry, sea moss, soursop bitters, black seed oil, collagen—the list continues, but you see the point. I feed my body healthy supplements, not medication (when there is an option).

Health is wealth so taking care of your body is an investment in yourself. I fought out of the binds of depression by moving my body at the gym several days a week. While I had to force myself to go after work, once I was there it always felt like a good choice. Eventually I disciplined myself to go early enough to go first thing in the morning before work. I started off walking as soon as my body allowed me to after treatment. Walking was my form of meditation. I listened to music or said positive affirmations declaring:

> I am light,
> I am healed,
> I am beautiful,

I am a child of God,
I am peace,
I am love,
I am enough.

My new normal actively shows love to myself with every action I take, feeding myself love language. Loving the woman in the mirror unapologetically. I am so committed to my growth that I am willing to say no without explanation nor guilt and yes without fear. My new normal is being comfortable being uncomfortable. My new normal is creating a life I have always dreamed of living. I know I can be strong, but can I be tender? Can I live a soft and gentle existence without losing strength? Each day I find ways to vibrate with good energy.

> John 8:12 NIV: When Jesus spoke again to the people, he said "I am the light of the world. Whoever follows me will never walk in darkness but will have the light of life."

On the other side of the cancer battle during recovery, I struggled with my self-confidence. Growing up, I noticed how women with fair skin and long hair were favored. As children, we teased dark-skinned, "bald-headed" people. In recovery, I had to deal with thinning, slow-growing, sparse hair and darker skin tone—I had no choice. I reinvented myself by getting braids or weave sewn in to add length and texture. When negative thoughts came to my mind, I countered with words of positivity. I acknowledged all I am from the inside out as a reminder of who God created me to be. My exterior does not define my core. Proverbs 31:30 has a verse for such an idea: "Charm is deceptive, and beauty is fleeting; but a woman who fears the LORD is to be praised."

I have become an advocate for other women recently diagnosed with breast cancer. Several of my friends, colleagues and relatives were diagnosed after me, and I immediately jumped into gear. I shared my experiences, my suggestions for making important changes in diet and life. I prayed with them and for them. I regularly check on them because we are united in our common ordeal. I applied for an Employer Identification Number to begin a foundation for Triple Negative Breast Cancer. My desire is to be a supporter and advocate for those going through Triple Negative Breast Cancer, which specifically impacts Black and Brown people at a higher rate and very aggressively. I began speaking publicly as a breast cancer survivor, and I plan to join breast cancer research in hopes of finding a cure.

> Hebrews 11:1 NIV: Now faith is confidence in what we hope for and assurance about what we do not see.

If you are reading this during any storms, like the ones I endured or others, I am sending you love and my prayers. Seek therapy if you have not done so already. God, therapy, and good friends saved my life many times. I stand with you to heal all the places you hurt. I stand with you letting go of vices and addictions that drain your power and block your release from the storm. You need a clear mind to free yourself from bonds. How do you show yourself that you love yourself? Set boundaries to protect your peace. Don't hurt your heart with people who are not genuine in their love for you. It hurts to walk away, but it will hurt more to stay. Pray to God for discernment. Fix your eyes on the joy that is possible in front of you. Could it be going back to school, learning a new hobby, discovering a new insight? Use your God-given gifts to make the world better.

As I write, my hands ache from neuropathy caused by chemo. The pain can be severe, and my hands often stiffen. Despite this, I remain committed to doing my best each day. Some days are harder, and sometimes I feel overwhelmed with sadness and cry. The feelings of grief over the person I was before cancer. Dealing with daily aches, pains, and neuropathy is tough. I usually stay positive, but sometimes sadness takes over. I rarely show it, as I prefer to keep it together with others. That takes a lot out of me in doing so which is why I usually stay home until I have enough energy to persistently push through my pains, physically and emotionally.

While scrolling Instagram one day, I heard Tabatha & Chance Brown speaking about purpose. Tabatha mentioned a minister who shared a story about all of us meeting with God in heaven before coming to Earth and mutually agreeing on our purpose. God has sent us to our parents on Earth to fulfill our purpose on Earth as it is in Heaven, just like it says in the Lord's Prayer: "Thy will be done on Earth as it is in Heaven." This confirmed so much to me and removed the guilt I felt over my babies being born as preemies with health complications, about being raped, about being the fault of any pain for someone else. Whatever has happened is a part of divine destiny.

> Psalm 46:10 KJV: Be still and know that I am God: I will be exalted among the heathen, I will be exalted in the earth.

I finally reached the acceptance part of my traumas, where I see clearly what happened and I have healed from it. Accepting is loving myself more each day on purpose. I am embracing how I show up in this world. I see my beauty in the presence of God in me, as he tells me I cannot save anyone but myself, and he will help me. I learned healing isn't about getting back to who I was before and not to rush, it's about embracing the new me that survived many storms. I still help people because I love doing so, however, I now have boundaries. It's challenging most days as I navigate this new space, but I remind myself it's not a race and my only competition is myself.

Writing this book is part of my purpose. Despite the loneliness of writing, God assigned it to me many times. Once, in 2003, I rode the Green Line train to work, and a lady I never met before said she was a prophetess. God told her to tell me I would write a book to help others heal from my own experiences. I didn't believe anything was unique about my life, so why bother writing a book? Since then, people have echoed that idea—write a book—and I heard but did not fully understand. Finally, the message was crystal clear during my battle. I needed to do what God purposed of me. I had to live my life yet separate myself enough from it to see what it all meant for the sake of helping others. I am grateful to all who understood on some level the purpose, even if we never spoke of it as such. They gave me the space and grace to fulfill my purpose.

> Jeremiah 29:11: For I know the plans I have for you, declares the Lord, plans to prosper
> you and not to harm you, plans to give
> you hope and a future.

MAKING FAITH MOVES

- This life does not promise only sunshine.
- If one lives long enough, many storms will come.
- The landscapes of our lives are not always flat and easy to walk.
- There are valleys that seem endless, and mountains that exhaust the climber.
- It's easy to look for ways around every challenge — to avoid pain, discomfort, or risk. But it always comes down to personal choices:
- What do we choose to accept? What do we choose to reject?

- Remember this — everything we choose to surround ourselves with has a greater purpose.
- Even the valleys where we stand during storms.
- Even the mountains we climb where we lose sight of the trail.
- There are always hidden markers waiting to guide us — toward healing, toward clarity, toward our ultimate destination.
- As you write in your journal, write down all the characteristics you love about yourself.
- Be your biggest cheerleader — but don't become egotistical.
- Spread love to all — but don't let anyone harm you.
- Stay informed — but don't overwhelm yourself as you grow and evolve.
- There is an art to being wise.
- It includes knowing:
- Who to ignore,
- When to move on,
- Where to leave what no longer serves you,
- And having the discernment to know what you can and cannot carry.
- Some people are not your assignment.
- People will try to convince you; you're not a good person when they can no longer take advantage of you.
- Be patient with yourself while things are still unfolding.
- I'm no longer interested in complicated relationships that require constant explanation.

- I will not shrink myself to make others comfortable — and if I'm "too much" for someone, I will not apologize.
- I celebrate my individuality and give myself permission to live a big life.
- This book is a record of my journey — a testament to how faith carried me through.
- It is not a blueprint.
- Your life will not look like mine.
- Your lessons will come differently.
- Your purpose is uniquely yours.
- But what I offer here are the markers I've encountered, the wisdom I've gathered, the emotions I've embraced, and the pain that shaped me into the person I needed to become.
- And I'm still becoming.
- You are too. We are not alone in this search — for ourselves, for each other, for meaning in all we survive.
- Discover what is inside you.
- Be free of every traumatic experience that ever convinced you to hide your true self. Stand tall in your worth. Own your healing.
- Make Faith Moves — every day, in your own purposeful way.
- No matter what.

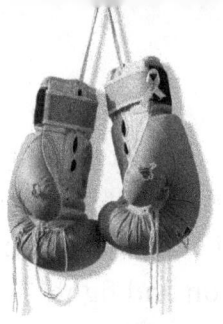

EPILOGUE BY JOSEPH L. REED

A JOURNEY OF LOVE, FAITH, AND STRENGTH FROM A HUSBAND'S PERSPECTIVE

Hello, world.

After reading Cassandra's story, I'm almost certain it will stir a wide range of emotions—some sad, some joyful, others uplifting and even surprising. I can personally attest to this, because from the first day I met her, she became my best friend. We instantly clicked and have since shared all those emotions together. That's just the kind of person she is—someone who brings out parts of you that you didn't even know were there.

Cassandra is rare—genuine, unique, and truly one of a kind. And allow me to introduce myself. As I mentioned, she's not only my best friend, but also my spouse and life partner. Today, I want to take you on a road trip into the mindset of a loving husband who also became her caretaker.

Please bear with me as I try to paint this picture. It's hard for me to write without getting emotional.

I remember the day like it was yesterday. I had just come home from work and saw my best friend crying. She told me she had discovered a lump in her breast and had gone for testing. I could see the fear in her eyes. Without hesitation, I dropped everything, held her tight, and told her, "Baby, don't worry. Gods got us. It's time to put the gloves on and fight." I already knew in my heart what we were facing.

I tried to be strong, to be her rock—but the emotions overwhelmed me. I cried with her. I had to. Like I said, Cassandra brings those emotions out of you. But even through the tears, I reassured her that everything was going to be okay—with prayer, faith, and grace.

Once we calmed down, we knew we had to act fast. She called her doctor right away and asked about the next steps. Her doctor provided a list of treatment centers and told us that it was going to be a journey—but it was one we could win. Because we caught it early, and with modern medicine, there was hope.

Now imagine seeing your best friend, the person you love most—completely broken, as if she had lost someone. I knew right then that my priorities were about to change. I was going to do everything in my power to help her get back to 100%.

We chose to start treatment at the Cancer Treatment Center. Yes, in case it isn't clear by now, I'm talking about breast cancer, the second deadliest disease after heart disease.

From that moment on, everything became "we." We were in this together. I promised her she wouldn't fight alone.

When the results came back, we learned it was stage 2B breast cancer. The treatment plan: 25 rounds of radiation, 16 rounds of chemotherapy, and multiple surgeries. It was overwhelming, especially when you're facing something so unfamiliar and terrifying.

As chemo began, new challenges arose. Cassandra experienced shortness of breath and, at times, couldn't walk. I had to get her a wheelchair. We were traveling miles back and forth to the center—sometimes daily—while I was still working 12- to 16-hour shifts at the steel mill, paying bills, and maintaining our home.

It was exhausting—physically, emotionally, spiritually. But giving up was never an option.

We both had sleepless nights. Still, I stayed committed to the promise I made to her. Everything else in life became secondary. I knew I had to lean on my faith. I prayed every day, sometimes three or four times a day. God became my best friend too. Prayer became second nature. And even when I doubted whether He was listening, I kept talking to Him. I poured out my heart, and eventually, my mind followed.

Then we faced another blow. The shortness of breath and difficulty walking turned out to be from a mass on her heart, caused by the chemo port. Another surgery. Another scare. Another moment where my faith was tested. But still, I held on. I reminded myself: God will never give you more than you can bear.

This trial revealed a strength in me I didn't know I had. It also showed me the man God was shaping me to become.

Eventually, Cassandra's breathing and ability to walk improved. But cancer doesn't stop throwing punches.

She lost her hair and a significant amount of weight. For anyone who knows my wife, you know how much she loves her hair. But she rocked her bald head with confidence. I offered to shave mine too, but she told me, "Bae, you don't need to do that. It's okay." Still, I assured her that she was beautiful—bald head and all.

We continued treatments, surrounded by an amazing team of doctors, nurses, and staff. And through it all, Cassandra kept her light. Her glow never faded. She walked into every room and lit it up—spreading positivity not just to me, but to everyone around her. Even in her weakest moments, she made others feel strong.

Once chemotherapy and radiation were done, we found out another surgery would be necessary. Still holding onto faith, we proceeded with genetic testing — and it revealed that Sandy carried the gene for ovarian cancer. That meant another major procedure. I was devastated. It felt like too much. But I reminded myself that God was still working — and He wouldn't have brought us this far just to leave us here.

My best friend — my wife — made the courageous decision to remove both breasts instead of just the tumor. She underwent a double mastectomy followed by reconstructive surgery. One of those surgeries lasted twelve hours. We were blessed with an incredible surgeon, Dr. Liu.

I was allowed to be nearby as Sandy prepared for surgery, but not by her side — and that was hard. Not being able to sit with her during that moment broke something open in me. I needed a moment to gather myself. So, I found a quiet bar, ordered a good bourbon, lit a cigar, and waited for the call that would change everything.

Throughout the night, my phone didn't stop ringing. Friends of Sandy's called not just to check on her, but to check on me. That's the kind of person she is — always thinking of others, always putting someone before herself. I updated her circle with each piece of news I received. Their love and support reminded me how truly blessed we are to have a community that surrounds us with such care.

Eventually, the call came. Surgery was successful. They told me when I could see her the next morning.

When I picked her up, she was in pain. And seeing her like that broke my heart — but I knew it was part of the healing. From then on, we followed a strict schedule of rest and recovery. If you know my wife, you know she doesn't sit still — not for a minute — but we made it work. I cooked, cleaned, did laundry, and helped her with anything she needed. Even bathing her. None of it mattered to me. I had a promise to keep to my best friend.

As we approached the end of her treatment journey, things started to look up. I won't lie—I was burnt out. But I was prepared to fight with her to the very end, no matter what the cost.

Little by little, things began to feel normal again. Friends and family stopped by often, offering help, encouragement, and love — something they still do to this day.

And now, I'm beyond proud to say:

Sandy has been cancer-free for four years.

We stay on schedule with our bi-annual checkups, doing our part, and trusting God with the rest.

This is more than just a cancer story. It's a story of love, loyalty, and faith. A story of what it means to walk through fire with your best friend and still come out glowing.

We're still on this journey, but I thank God every day for Cassandra—for her strength, her spirit, and the way she continues to inspire everyone she meets.

This journey has taught me so much. To never doubt God. To always believe — even when it's hard. To never question the strength that lives in us. And most of all:

Always make faith moves.

J. Reed

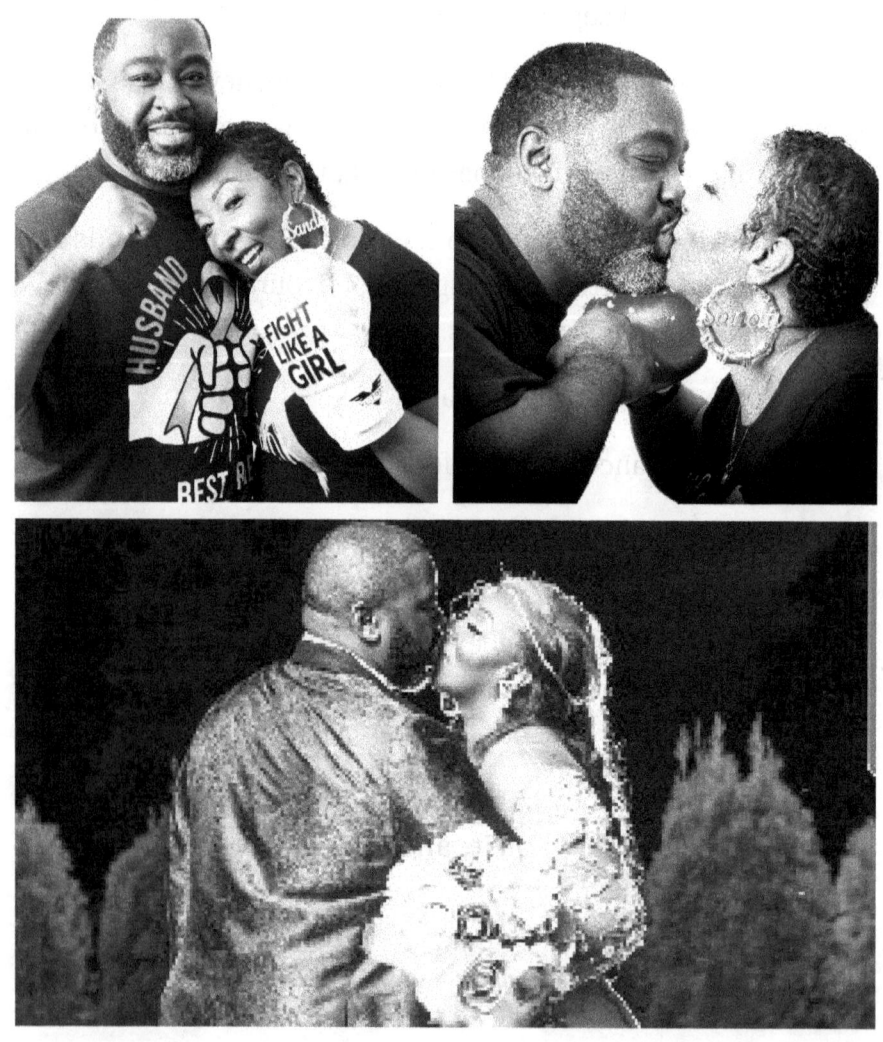

ACKNOWLEDGEMENTS

First, giving glory to God who is the head of my life. God put this book on my spirit decades ago and I refused to believe that I had a story worth sharing. God kept giving me a testimony. It was when I was in my bed fighting through side effects from chemotherapy God reminded me to write this book. I surrendered in that moment regardless of any negative backlash I would receive in sharing my story. This story is my honest recollection of my life events that showed how I personally used my faith to get through the traumas that I shared.

God blessed me with a good man Savannah, lol. My husband, Joe, thank you for your patience, your love, your spirit, your hard work, your smile when I needed it, your strong arms for me to collapse in. You came into my life at a time when I was drained and tired as a mother. I had been a single mother for so long, doing it all on my own and when you came into my life you took the time to show me what a real man does, you removed my burdens. You saw through my tough exterior and broke down my walls I had up towards men. I felt depleted as a woman taking care of everyone but myself, you saw me and empowered me and loved me completely. Thank you for helping me raise our children, helping me earn my MBA, helping me battle breast cancer and supporting me through writing this book. There are no words I can fully express to capture how much I adore you, respect you, honor you and appreciate you. You are amazing and I am your biggest fan.

I am blessed to have four boys and a girl. My first borns Twins, Neon (born 2 minutes before Deon), thank you for your love, support and teaching me patience and kindness. I know watching me battle cancer hurt you to your core, however you pushed through it with prayer.

You always have led with your heart and take care of people even before taking care of yourself. I appreciate your love and support, and I love you endlessly. Deon, my Don cheche, I nicknamed you that as a baby because you always had boss energy. You came into the world proclaiming your presence and letting everyone know you don't need any help. You taught me grit and humbleness. I appreciate you and I adore you always. I became a mother because of you both. Thank you for choosing me. Thank you for believing in me and giving me the honor to raise you, we grew up together. Thank you for showing me that I am worthy of that title.

My one and only girl, JaNiya, you came into my life and helped me smooth out my rough parts, to become a little softer. Thank you for teaching me gentleness and trusting me with your love, your heart and your father. You are the daughter I always wanted. I enjoy our moments together talking and sharing our future goals with our warm hugs. Watching you evolve into the young woman you have become has been an absolute joy. I am proud of you, your hard work and ambition. I love you forever. To my Zion, you are a silent weapon, you don't say much but when you do you speak with integrity. You are a natural born leader with honesty and devotion to your goals. I named you after the city of Zion where people went to pray. You are a safe space for everyone you love. You encouraged me through my battle at the young age of thirteen, you weren't selfish about your needs like people speak of typical teenagers. You are not typical. You woke up daily, checked on me, making sure I ate and protected my peace from anything or anyone that could cause me any stress. I love you eternally.

My Jojo, I know I nicknamed you that as a little boy and you have now grown into a teenager with a big heart and so much talent. It has been a distinct privilege to witness your development and support your growth. I hold each of you in high regard and commend your character, integrity, kindness, accountability, and respectfulness. Regardless of future circumstances, please know that my continued love, encouragement and support will remain unwavering.

My parents! I was blessed with great parents. My mother and father were both hard workers. I learned how to work and play from them. I saw how a woman should carry herself from watching my mother. I saw how a man should treat me from how my father loved me. I appreciate how you both cared for me during my cancer battle. My father dropped everything and traveled from Arizona to care for me and my family. My mother packed a bag and came to stay at our home whenever me and Joe asked. Everything I do, I try to make you guys proud of me. I hear your voice in my decisions as I move in this world. Thank you both. I love you both so much and always will honor, respect and value you for teaching me I can do anything I put my mind to achieve.

Thank you, Sugarplum, for agreeing to adding your voice in the form of the foreword to my book. Thank you for agreeing to speak at my wedding reception. I appreciate everything you add to my life and for always allowing me to only show up as myself without explanation. You hold me accountable without losing our connection. You protect me. I am so proud of the woman you have become; I have watched you grow up as my baby cousin and become my sister in every sense of the word. I was there to watch you graduate from high school and college. I am proud of you. I love and adore you endlessly.

E.knox, baby bro and my twin. I appreciate you agreeing to be the MC at my wedding reception on short notice. It was my pleasure to stand up and speak at your wedding. Thank you and Sammy for checking on me, coming to see me from AZ and allowing us to stay at your home when we visited AZ. Our connection means the world to me. We identify with each other across geographic locations and no matter how much time elapses between us communicating.

My siblings; Alonzo, Jeanette, Elijah, Samantha, Ebony. my cousins; Terry, Jobe Jr, Alex, Earl, Necee, Teneshia (my Cake), Stevie, Tinesha (my Petunia), Marcus, Hollis, Aireale, Nicole, Trina, Shaquela, LaToya, Ida, Dwyane, Carol, Shelby, Joe, Georgia, Carrie Joe, Robbie, Kimberly, Stafford, Tracey, Felicia, Charles, Evelyn, Joyce, Mike, Darien, Demi, Selina, Terrell, Stephon, Karen, Karon, Destiny, Rakim, Dominiq, Danielle. my aunts; Arnitha, Renee, Carol, Bettye, Sharon, Loretta. my uncles; Gregory, Anthony, Tony. My nieces; Simone, Sade, and my nephews; Selbie, Savon, Alonzo.

My sister friends, Maxine, Woodie, Nicole, Belinda, Phenia, Chanetha, Esha, Ketari, Jafrika, and Angel. Mommatine, Mama Vanessa. My childhood friends; Tonya, Chanita, Chakeesha, Hafeesa, Marayah, Kelle, James Williams, LaChanda, Tiffany, Purity, Felicia, Sir Lloyd, DJ, Starles. My friends since high school; Lisa, Kimmy, Sheri, Tekeia, Sheronda, Tiffany, Roxanne, RaMeka, Ta'Shara, Sheree, Camile, Daniel, Keith, Bruce, Lucas, Alicia, Tracy, Jaida, D'onshontia, Shonte, Marnita, Christina, Samuel, Jermeka, Q Sandifer, Tanara.

My friends since college; Kendis, Natasha, Lolita, Vexton, Anthony, Mica, Shay, Allison, Tylynn, DeShonka, Michelle, Nathaniel, Zeno, Lateef, Razelle, Ayanna. My colleagues and friends; Inez, Tawanda, Mimi, Elaine, Nevita, Roniece, Yvette, Cassandra, Annette, Tamica, Carla, June, Arlisa, BJ, Casey, Elodie. In-laws; Poppa Joe, Mama Pam Reed, Aunt Jackie, Nita, Aja, Charmaine, Brittany, Lelee, Simone, Chyna, Irish, Kyla, Antonio, Paula, Sandericka, Karen, Paul, Thelma, Odessa, Fredeja, Stevie, Shondra. To all the people's lives that have touched mine, we are forever connected no matter where we met; Amirius (God son/nephew), Jalisa (God daughter/niece), Galeca (niece), Jamesha (niece), Jaliya (niece), Sara (niece), Amar'yah (niece),

Shamir (nephew), Javair (nephew), Raquel (niece), Kina, Cortez (nephew), Dajuan (nephew), Aj (nephew), Karen, Toya, Andrea, Alana, Ebony, Aunt Shirley, Aunt Gertie, Aunt Tawanda, Aunt Marcia, Gloria, Kim, Doriece, Carl, Dr. Scott-Terry and her entire office, Shanequa, Shar, Antoine, Reginald, Sherrye White, Shamara, Tonya Rodgers, Samantha, Jermaine, Rodney and family, Reed family, Chandler family, Cook family, Hudson family, Moore family.

To those who passed away on my journey, thank you all for watching over me, Great Grandma Flora, Grandma Janet, Sister, Clarence, Grandaddy Sonny, Uncle Jobe, my cousin Karen, Dominique, James, Eric, Aunt Adrian, Uncle Kimble, Ms. Nancy, Momma Francine, Mama Helen, Michelle G, Willie G., Mama Dot, Mama Pam, Hernando.

I am eternally grateful to you all. If I fail to mention anyone, please charge it to my head and not my heart you all know I am suffering from chemo brain and menopause. I love you all on purpose 12

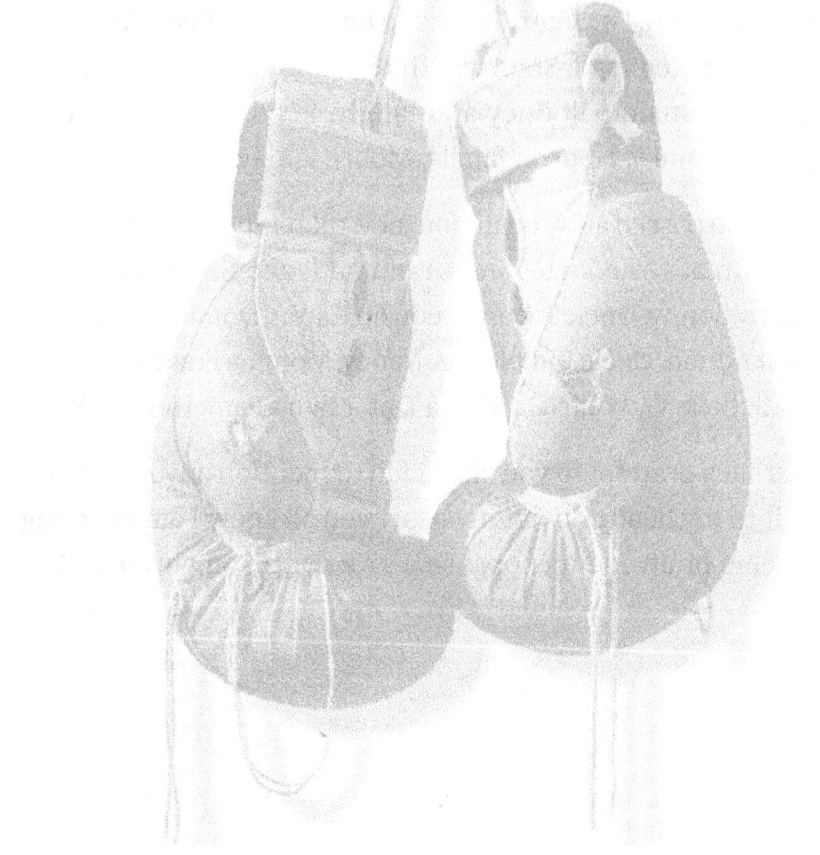

www.ingramcontent.com/pod-product-compliance
Lightning Source LLC
Chambersburg PA
CBHW070531090426
42735CB00013B/2944